R. A. Witthaus

A laboratory guide in urinalysis and toxicology

R. A. Witthaus

A laboratory guide in urinalysis and toxicology

ISBN/EAN: 9783742805874

Manufactured in Europe, USA, Canada, Australia, Japa

Cover: Foto ©Lupo / pixelio.de

Manufactured and distributed by brebook publishing software
(www.brebook.com)

R. A. Witthaus

A laboratory guide in urinalysis and toxicology

A

LABORATORY GUIDE

IN

URINALYSIS AND TOXICOLOGY

BY

R. A. WITTHAUS, Á.M., M.D.

PROFESSOR OF CHEMISTRY AND PHYSICS IN THE MED. DEPT. UNIVERSITY OF THE
CITY OF NEW YORK ; PROFESSOR OF CHEMISTRY AND TOXICOLOGY IN THE MED.
DEPT. UNIVERSITY OF VERMONT ; PROFESSOR OF CHEMISTRY AND TOXICOL-
OGY IN THE MED. DEPT. UNIVERSITY OF BUFFALO ; PROFESSOR OF PHAR-
MACEUTICAL CHEMISTRY IN THE DEPT. OF PHARMACY, UNIVERSITY
OF BUFFALO ; CHEMIST TO THE CITY OF BUFFALO ; CHEMIST TO
THE N. Y. STATE DAIRY COMMISSIONER ; MEMBER OF THE
AMERICAN CHEMICAL SOCIETY, AND OF THE CHEMICAL
SOCIETIES OF PARIS AND BERLIN, ETC., ETC.

NEW YORK
WILLIAM WOOD & COMPANY
57 & 58 LAFAYETTE PLACE
1886

PRESS OF
STETTINER, LAMBERT & CO.,
129 & 131 CROSBY ST.,
NEW YORK.

CONTENTS.

URINALYSIS AND TOXICOLOGY.

GENERAL RULES FOR WORKING.

1. There is a place for everything, into which it must be put *immediately* after use.

2. The reagent bottles must be kept upon the shelves in the order of their numbers, and with the labels outward.

3. In replenishing reagent bottles from stock, fill them only half full.

4. If the reagent in any bottle become cloudy, filter it.

5. *Do not lay the stopper of the bottle upon the table.* Remove it from the bottle by grasping it between the little and ring fingers of the left hand, and hold it there, pointing outward from the back of the hand, until replaced in the bottle.

6. In liquid tests, use about two cent. of the liquid to be tested in a test-tube; not more unless so directed.

7. Add the reagent in small quantity at first, and stop when the desired end is attained.

8. Prevent the last drop adhering to the lip of the bottle from flowing down its side, by catching it upon the stopper or upon the *clean* lip of the test-tube.

9. A separate portion of the original substance or liquid is to be used for each test, except when otherwise directed.

10. Before trying a reaction, read the description through, and then follow the directions literally. *Should the result not be that described, ask for an explanation.*

11. Let each piece of apparatus be clean before being put into its place, and let everything be in its place before you leave.

ABBREVIATIONS.

The following abbreviations are used in the text, and will be found convenient by the student in taking notes:

ppt. = precipitate	pt.—pts. = part—parts
pptn. = precipitation	dil. = dilute
sol. = soluble	cent. = centimetres
insol. = insoluble	gtt. = drops
soln. = solution	sp. gr. = specific gravity
cc. = cubic centimetre	con. = concentrated
L. = litre	gm. = gram.

The formula *of the reagent* always applies to its solution, except where otherwise specified.

Metric weights and measures, and the centigrade thermometric scale are used throughout.

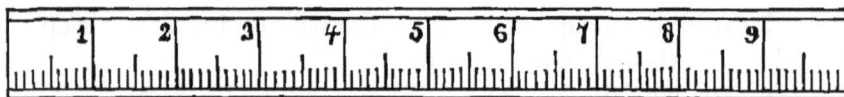

One decimetre.

QUALITATIVE ANALYSIS OF URINE.

PHYSICAL CHARACTERS.

Quantity.

1. Collect all urine passed by the patient during twenty-four hours, and measure in a cylindrical graduate (Fig. 1), divided into cubic centimetres.

Normal = 1,000 *to* 1,500 *cc.*

All examinations of urine should be made with samples of the mixed urine of twenty-four hours, unless otherwise directed.

Color.

2. Put 100 cc. urine (filtered if cloudy) into a beaker of 6 to 7 centimetres diameter; look through it at the light from a window, and compare the color observed with the color plate. Record this, by using the numbers of the colored squares, as *free color.* Add 5 cc. HCl to the urine; stir, let stand four hours, compare color as before, and record as *total color.*

Odor.

3. Note whether the odor is natural or "urinous," or "ammoniacal," "like violets," or otherwise peculiar.

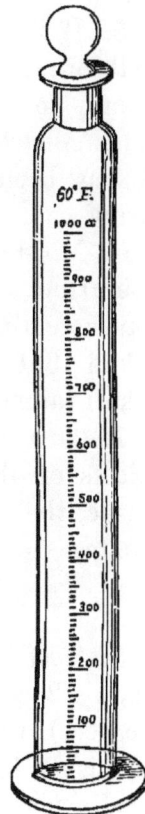

FIG. 1.

Reaction.

4. Put some of the urine into a porcelain capsule; dip into it a piece of red and a piece of blue litmus paper. If the blue paper turn red, the reaction is *acid*. If the red paper turn blue, the reaction is *alkaline*. If the colors remain unchanged, the reaction is *neutral*.

5. If the reaction be found to be alkaline, it remains to determine whether the alkalinity is due to fixed or volatile alkali, to carbonates or phosphates. These determinations must be made with the urine so soon as possible after it has been voided, and, preferably, with the morning urine.

6. Moisten one-half of a piece of red litmus paper with the urine, and hang it up to dry. If, after drying, the paper retain its blue color, the alkalinity is due to fixed alkali ; but if the paper return to its original red, to volatile alkali (ammonia).

7. To a portion of the urine in a test tube add a slight excess of HCl, and warm, if necessary; if effervescence ensue, the alkalinity is due to carbonates ; if not, to phosphates.

Specific Gravity.

8. Test the urinometer (which should not be smaller than 12 centimetres in length, and divided into single degrees) with the solutions of known specific gravity furnished in the laboratory for that purpose, making the readings as directed in § 9, and note the error in different parts of the scale. The differences from the true readings are to be noted on the box, and added or subtracted, as the error is minus or plus, in all subsequent readings.

9. To use the urinometer : The cylinder should be of the shape shown in Fig. 2, without pouring-lip, of such depth that the urinometer may be completely immersed,

and of a diameter double that of the wide part of the urinometer.

Hold the cylinder in an inclined position, and pour into
it urine to within 2 centimetres of the
top. Set it upright, float the urinometer in the urine, and add more urine
until the level "heaps" above the
rim of the cylinder. Now bring the
eye to about the level of the top of
the cylinder, and, seeing that the urinometer does not touch the wall of
the cylinder, read off the specific
gravity at the *highest* point where the
liquid, drawn up by capillary attrac-
tion, cuts the graduation of the urinometer (A, Fig. 2).

10. The temperature at which the
gravity should be determined is 60°
F. (= 15°.4 Cent.). If the urine be
of a different temperature, cool it by
immersing the vessel in cold water,
or warm it until 60° is reached.

Corrections for variations of temperature cannot be accurately made
in the case of a liquid of such com-
plex and varying composition as the
urine.

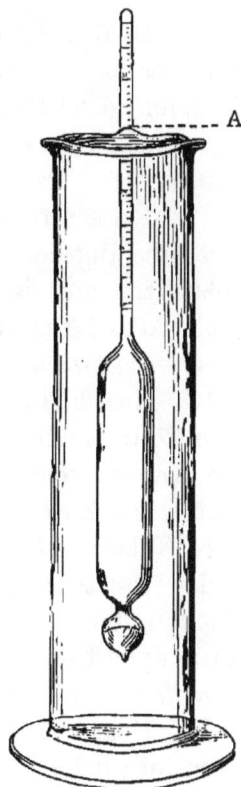

FIG. 2.

CHEMICAL CHARACTERS—COMPOSITION.

Normal Constituents.

N. B.—Obviously a qualitative examination of the urine
for its normal constituents is never practised by the phy-
sician. The student is required to test for the more important of these substances, partly that he may be able to

recognize them elsewhere, but principally to afford practice in the methods of manipulation and observation.

Mineral and Organic Substances.

11. Heat a slip of clean platinum foil in the flame until it ceases to color the latter yellow. Place upon the foil a fragment of chalk, and heat in the flame. The chalk does not blacken or volatilize. Chalk is a *fixed mineral substance.*

12. Place a fragment of NH_4Cl in the bottom of a dry test-tube and heat it cautiously. It does not blacken, but volatilizes, and is deposited in its original form upon the cool part of the tube. Ammonium chloride is a *volatile mineral substance.*

13. Heat a fragment of starch upon a slip of clean platinum foil; it blackens (after burning), and on continuing the heat the coal gradually disappears, and nothing is left. Starch is a *fixed organic substance.*

14. Place a fragment of benzoic acid in the bottom of a dry test tube and heat it cautiously. It does not blacken, but volatilizes, and is deposited in its original form upon the cool part of the tube. Benzoic acid is a *volatile organic substance.*

15. Heat a piece of dry albumin upon the slip of platinum foil; it burns, blackens, and also gives off an odor of burnt horn. Albumin is a *nitrogenized, colloid organic substance.*

16. Heat a fragment of urea upon the clean platinum foil; it neither burns nor does it give an odor of burnt horn, but fuses, gives off an odor of ammonia, and finally disappears. Urea is a *crystalloid, nitrogenized organic substance.*

N. B.—It will be seen from the above that organic and mineral substances which are not capable of volatilizing unchanged may be distinguished from each other by the blackening and burning of the former when heated. Volatile organic and mineral substances cannot, however, be distinguished in this way. The albuminoid substances may be further recognized by the odor which they emit on burning, while many other nitrogenized organic substances give off ammonia when heated, and behave precisely as do certain ammoniacal salts.

Chlorides.

17. Put some of the liquid to be tested into two test-tubes,* add to each gtt. 5 $AgNO_3$—a white ppt.† is produced. To one of the test-tubes add NH_4HO and agitate —the ppt. redissolves completely. To the other test-tube add HNO_3 and agitate—the ppt. does not redissolve.

Phosphates.

18. Add $AgNO_3$ to the liquid in two test-tubes—a yellow ppt. is produced. Add NH_4HO to the liquid in one test-tube and NO_3H to that in the other, and agitate—the ppt. in each redissolves.

19. Add magnesia mixture ‡—a white, crystalline ppt. is formed. Add HCl—the ppt. redissolves.

Sulphates.

20. Add $BaCl_2$—a white ppt. is formed. Add HCl to strongly acid reaction—the ppt. does not redissolve.

---

* The student is referred to the General Rules, p. 1, which he should hold in mind.

† See abbreviations, p. 2.

‡ Made by dissolving 11 pts. $MgCl_2$ and 28 pts. NH_4Cl in 130 pts. NH_4HO, adding 70 pts. dil. NH_4HO and filtering after two days.

Urea.

21. To a moderately concentrated cold soln. of urea in a watch glass add colorless HNO_3 in equal volume—immediately, or after a few moments, crystals of nitrate of urea (Fig. 3) separate.

22. To a few drops of a soln. of urea upon a watch glass add a few gtt. of Millon's reagent,* and heat—a yellow color, changing to red is produced. A somewhat similar appearance is produced with albumins.

23. Heat a fragment of urea in a dry test-tube until, after having fused, it is converted into an opaque, white solid; let cool; add about 1 cent. KHO and gtt. 2 of a very dilute soln. $CuSO_4$,—a pale rose-red color. This test, known as the *"biuret reaction,"* produces a similar appearance with peptones. See § 39.

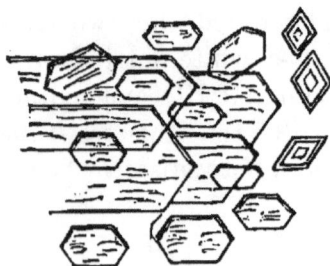

Fig. 3.

Uric Acid.

24. Moisten the solid in a porcelain capsule with a few gtt. HNO_3; heat on the water bath until dry; cool; add NH_4HO—a brilliant red color appears, which fades after a few moments. This is known as the *"murexid test."*

Abnormal Constituents.

PROTEIDS—ALBUMINOIDS.

Before testing for albuminoids, the urine must be separated from all solid particles, must be rendered perfectly

* Made by dissolving 1 pt. Hg. in 2 pts. strong HNO_3 over the water bath, diluting with 2 pts. H_2O and decanting after four hours.

clear and transparent; this is accomplished by the process of

Filtration.

The apparatus required for this purpose consists of a funnel and support for the same, a vessel to receive the *filtrate* (*i. e.*, the liquid which passes through the filter), a wash bottle, stirring-rod, and *filters*.

The funnel (Fig. 4) should be selected by testing with a piece of card-board cut with an angle of 60° (A Fig. 4), which should exactly fit it, and should have the point of the stem ground off at an angle.

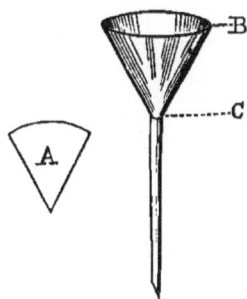 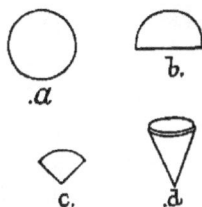 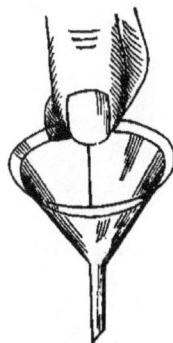

Fig. 4.   FIG. 5.   FIG. 6.

The filters are discs of porous paper manufactured for the purpose (filter paper). The radius of the disc selected should be somewhat less than the length of the sloping side of the funnel from rim to shoulder (B-C Fig. 4). The filter must not project above the rim of the funnel.

25. Take a filter (*a*, Fig. 5) of suitable size and fold it across a diameter (*b*, Fig. 5), fold it again over a radius at right angles to the first diameter (*c*, Fig. 5), open the paper out into a conical bag by separating one thickness of the paper from the other three (*d*, Fig. 5). The filter is then adjusted in the funnel and pressed against its side with the *dry finger* until it fits closely. Now, holding the.

filter and funnel so that the nail of the fore-finger is pressed against the upper end of one of the folds (Fig. 6), moisten the paper by directing upon it a jet of water from the orifice *a* of the wash bottle (Fig. 7), produced by blowing gently into the tube *b*.

26. Support the funnel containing the wetted filter over

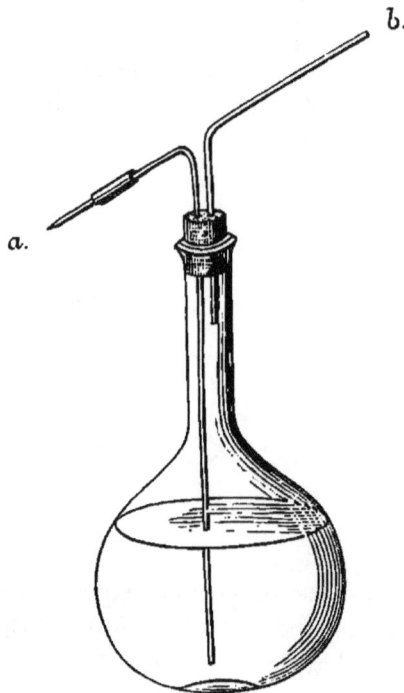

FIG. 7.

the vessel destined to receive the filtrate (if a flask or test-tube be used for this purpose, no other support is needed), and pour the liquid to be filtered into the filter, allowing it to flow along the stirring-rod, held as shown in Fig 8, in successive portions until it has passed through; never, however, adding liquid in greater quantity than to within two to three millimetres of the edge of the filter.

27. It frequently happens that urine does not yield a clear filtrate by simple filtration.   When this is the case,

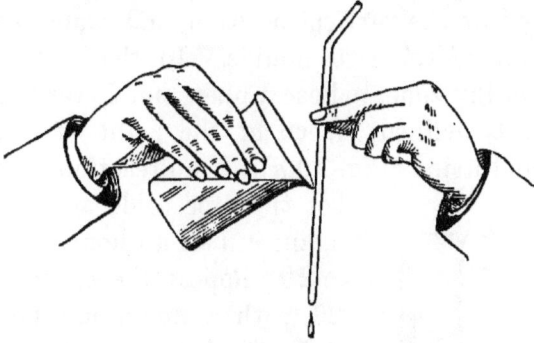

Fig. 8.

add to the turbid filtrate enough KHO to communicate a distinctly alkaline reaction, and a few gtt. of magnesia mixture, warm slightly and filter again through a fresh filter.

Albumin.

28. *Heller's test.*—Put about 2 cent. HNO_3 into a

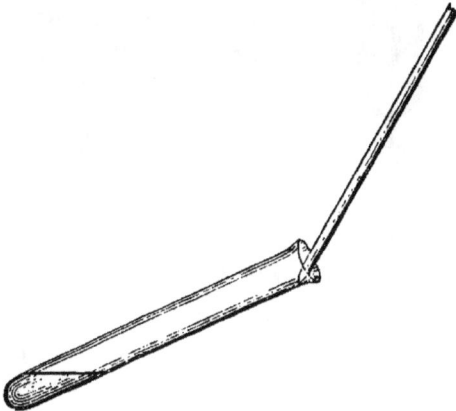

Fig. 9.

test-tube.   Fill a pipette with the filtered urine.   Hold the test-tube at a small angle to the horizontal, and allow the

urine to flow *slowly* from the pipette (whose upper end
has been roughened by the file) upon the surface of the
nitric acid (Fig 9). Remove the pipette, turn the test-tube
cautiously into the vertical position, and examine the point
of junction of the two liquids. In the presence of albumin a milky zone, whose upper and lower borders are
both sharply defined, is seen *at* the point of junction of
the acid and urine (Fig. 10 *a*). If no reaction be observed,
set the tube aside and examine it
again in half an hour.

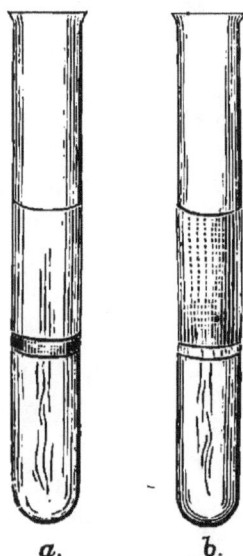

Fɪɢ. 10.

29. Repeat the testing, as in §
28, with a non-albuminous urine.
A band of deeper coloration is observed at the point of junction of
the two liquids; this is not to be
confounded with the milky zone
observed with albuminous urine.

30. Repeat the testing, as in §
28, using a urine containing an excess of urates, but no albumin.
A white zone is observed *above* the
point of junction of the liquids,
whose lower border may be sharply
defined, but whose upper border
fades off gradually into the layer
of urine, the whole of which may
become turbid (Fig. 10 *b*).

31. *Heat and Nitric Acid test.*—Determine the reaction
of the urine. If it be alkaline, add acetic acid cautiously until it shows a *faintly* acid reaction with blue litmus paper.
Fill a test-tube to within 2–3 cent. of the top with the
acidulated urine, and, holding the test-tube by the bottom,
heat the upper portion of the liquid *nearly to boiling*. An
opalescence, cloudiness, or coagulum is formed, according

to the amount of albumin present. Now add slowly 15 to
30 gtt. of concentrated HNO_3; the ppt. does not dimin-
ish (it may increase) in amount.

32. Apply heat, as in § 31, to a sample of the alkaline
albuminous urine, without acidulating. No reaction is
observed.

33. Apply heat, as in § 31, to another sample of the
urine, to which an excess of acetic acid has been added.
No reaction is observed.

34. Apply the test, as directed in § 31, to a sample of
urine containing no albumin, but containing an excess of
earthy phosphates. An appearance similar to that observed in the case of the albuminous urine is obtained; but
on addition of HNO_3, the ppt. redissolves and the liquid
becomes transparent.

34a. *Picric Acid test.*—Float some of the *clear* urine on
acetic acid as in Heller's test. If any cloudiness be observed at the junction of the two liquids, treat a larger
quantity of the urine with acetic acid to acid reaction, and
filter. Pour about 7 cent. of the *clear* filtrate, or of the
clear urine, which gives no cloudiness when floated on
acetic acid, into a test-tube; float upon its surface about
2 cent. of a saturated solution of picric acid and warm the
point where the two liquids come together. A cloudiness
at this point, which does not disappear when heat is applied, is evidence of the presence of albumin.

A cloudiness which *does* disappear on the application
of heat may be produced by alkaloids, urates, etc.

Paraglobulin.

35. Dilute the filtered urine, slightly acidulated with
acetic acid if necessary, with water to sp. gr. 1.002, and
pass through it a current of carbon dioxide. A cloudiness,

either on dilution or after treatment with CO_2, indicates the presence of paraglobulin.

Mucin.

36. Pour about 2 cent. of acetic acid into a test-tube, and float the clear urine upon its surface. A cloud, which usually appears only after standing a time, just above the line of contact of the liquids, shows the presence of mucin, provided it does not disappear on the application of heat.

Peptone.

37. Add soln. of neutral lead acetate to 500 cc. urine, until the ppt. no longer increases; filter. To the filtrate add acetic acid and a few gtt. of ferrocyanide of potassium soln.; if any cloudiness be produced, continue the addition of ferrocyanide soln. until the precipitate no longer increases, and filter.

38. To a portion of the last filtrate obtained as in § 37, add one-fifth its bulk of acetic acid and then an acid soln. of sodium phosphotungstate.* A cloudiness immediately, or after a few moments, indicates the presence of peptone.

39. To the remainder of the filtrate, § 37, add half its volume of strong HCl, and then phosphotungstate soln. to complete precipitation. Collect the ppt. on a filter as rapidly as possible, wash with 5% H_2SO_4 until the filtrate is colorless. Transfer the ppt. to a capsule and mix it thoroughly with powdered barium hydrate; add a little H_2O; warm fifteen minutes on the water bath, and filter. Add to a portion of the filtrate in a test-tube KHO soln. to strongly

---

* The phosphotungstate soln. is made by adding phosphoric acid to a boiling soln. of sodium-tungstate to acid reaction, cooling, adding acetic acid to strongly acid reaction, and filtering after twenty-four hours.

alkaline reaction, and then 1 gtt. of a dil. soln. of $CuSO_4$ A reddish-violet color indicates the presence of peptone. See § 23.

Glucose—Diabetic Sugar.*

40. If the urine contain albumin, this must be removed before testing for sugar. If the urine be not already acid, acidulate it with acetic acid. Heat the acid urine in a flask or beaker, and when it begins to boil, add 2 gtt. acetic acid and boil for half an hour, or until the albumin, which was at first disseminated throughout the liquid, has separated in flocks. Filter, and apply the following tests to the filtrate:

41. Urine containing sugar is *usually* of high sp. gr., pale in color, abundant in quantity, and sometimes has a sweetish odor.

42. *Moore's test.*—To the urine in two test-tubes add one-half bulk of KHO. Boil the contents of one tube for about a minute, and then compare its color with that of the other tube. A darkening of the boiled sample indicates the presence of sugar.

N. B.—In boiling a liquid in a test-tube, hold the tube by its upper end, between the thumb and forefinger, the mouth pointing over the forefinger and away from the person. Hold the bottom of the tube in the flame until small bubbles begin to rise through the liquid, then, and so long as the heating continues, prevent "bumping" of the contents by an oscillation of the tube, produced by rapidly alternating slight motions of pronation and supination of the hand.

---

* Glucose is considered as an abnormal constituent of the urine for clinical convenience. Strictly speaking, it is a normal constituent. It is constantly present, but in such minute quantity, that the tests, as usually applied, fail to reveal its presence so long as the quantity remains within the normal limits.

In cases where prolonged boiling is necessary, the tube may be held in a wooden clamp, or by passing around its upper part a folded strip of strong paper, whose ends are then grasped between the thumb and forefinger.

43. *Trommer's test.*—To the urine in a test-tube add 2 gtt. of a saturated soln. of $CuSO_4$ and a volume of KHO soln. equal to half that of the urine. Observe that the liquid is blue and transparent. Heat until the liquid *begins* to boil. The formation of a yellow or red ppt. indicates the presence of glucose.

44. Apply the test as described in § 43, using a urine containing a large amount of sugar. The liquid changes in color from blue to yellow, but no ppt. is produced.

45. Repeat the testing of the highly saccharine urine, adding gtt. 6 in place of gtt. 2 $CuSO_4$ soln., and allow the liquid to stand after boiling. The yellow or red ppt. is produced.

46. Repeat the test with the urine used in § 43, adding gtt. 6 $CuSO_4$ soln., and boiling for a longer time. A black or dark colored ppt. is produced.

N. B.—Trommer's test only shows that sugar is present when a *distinct yellow or red ppt.* is formed. A mere change of color, or the formation of a ppt. different from that described is not sufficient evidence of the presence of sugar. Therefore, in applying this test in practice, use only a small quantity of $CuSO_4$ soln. at first, and if in a first testing a change of color be observed, but no ppt., make a second testing, using an increased amount of $CuSO_4$.

47. *Boettger's test.*—Render the urine strongly alkaline by dissolving in it powdered Na_2CO_3. Put into two test-tubes about 3 cent. of the alkaline urine. To one test-tube add a very minute quantity of powdered subnitrate of bismuth, to the other as much powdered litharge. Boil the contents of the two tubes. If sugar be present, the bismuth powder becomes first gray and then black. The litharge is not blackened.

48. Repeat the test as in § 47 with a urine containing a sulphide or an organic compound containing sulphur, but no sugar. Both subnitrate and litharge are blackened.

49. *Mulder-Neubauer test.*—Dissolve in 2 cent. of the saccharine urine in a test-tube enough powdered Na_2CO_3 to give it a strongly alkaline reaction, and then enough solution of indigo-carmine to communicate a distinctly blue color. Heat the liquid to boiling with as little agitation as possible. The color changes from blue to green, to wine-red, to yellow. Allow the contents of the tube to cool, close the opening of the tube with the thumb, and agitate; the color changes back through wine-red and green to blue.

50. *Fermentation test.*—Take three beakers of about 70 cc. capacity, and label them A, B, and C. Fill A with the urine to be tested; B with a solution of glucose, and C with water. Put into each beaker some brewers' yeast, or some compressed yeast, and stir well. Fill a test-tube completely full from A. Close the opening of the tube with a cork of suitable size fastened on the short limb of a wire bent at right angles, in such a way that no air bubbles are inclosed. Immerse the end of the tube with the cork into the liquid in A, and remove the cork by means of the wire, taking care that no air enters the tube. Reverse test-tubes similarly filled from B and C in each of those beakers. Set the three beakers and tubes in a place whose temperature is about 25°, and after six hours observe whether gas have collected in any of the tubes. If the test-tubes A and B contain gas above the liquid, and C do not, the urine contains sugar. If A and C do not contain gas, and B do, the urine does not contain sugar. Under any other circumstances the yeast is unfit for use.

The purpose of A is to test the urine; that of B and C to guard against sources of error from the yeast itself.

51. *Fehling's test.*—Put about 2 cent. of Fehling's solution (see § 88) into a test-tube, and heat it to boiling. Examine the liquid carefully—standing with your back to the light, and, if possible, holding the tube in the direct rays of the sun—for any red specks or reddish reflections, which appear usually at the lower, curved part of the tube. If any red color be observed, the test solution has deteriorated and must be replaced by some which has been freshly mixed.

52. If the test solution have been found to be in proper condition, add to it 2 to 3 gtt. of the urine to be tested, and boil again. If no red color be now observed, add a further quantity of urine, and boil again. Continue this alternate addition of urine and boiling until a red or yellow ppt. is formed—in which case sugar is present—or until a bulk of urine equal to that of the test solution used has been added, without the appearance of a red ppt.— in which case sugar is absent.

N. B.—Fehling's solution is recommended as affording the most manageable and reliable test for sugar, provided the precautions mentioned in §§ 51 and 40 are observed. When the amount of sugar present is very small, the liquid retains its blue color; but when it is poured out of the tube, a red film is seen attached to the glass. If the quantity of sugar be great, the copper is completely precipitated, and the liquid decolorized.

Test-tubes which have been used for Fehling's and Trommer's tests may be cleaned with a little HNO_3.

Blood.

53. If the urine be alkaline, render it *faintly* acid with acetic acid. Heat to near boiling. The urine becomes lighter in color, and a dark colored coagulum is formed.

54. Add KHO to distinct alkaline reaction; heat nearly to boiling (do not boil). A red ppt. is produced.

55. To a few drops of the urine in a test-tube add a drop of freshly prepared tincture of guaiacum and a little ozonic ether (ether to which oxygenated water has been added) and agitate. The ether, which rises to the surface, is blue.

Or, shake together oil of turpentine and tincture of guaiac, add the urine in volume equal to that of the emulsion, shake gently, and allow to separate: a blue or greenish-blue color in the upper layer.

Bile.

Biliary Salts.

56. *Pettenkofer's test.*—Add to the urine in a test-tube 1 gtt. of a · solution of cane-sugar (1 : 3); hold the tube in an inclined position, and add H_2SO_4 in such a way that it forms a layer below the urine. In the presence of biliary acids, the urine becomes turbid, and immediately, or after a time, a purple-red band is formed at the junction of the two liquids, which gradually diffuse into one another, forming, after four to five hours, a homogeneous dark-purple liquid. The acid and urine must not be mixed.

57. Repeat the test, as in § 56, with urine containing albumin, but no biliary salts. The same reaction is produced.

58. Repeat the test, as in § 56, with urine containing morphia, but no biliary salts. The same reaction is produced.

59. As albumin, morphia, and a number of other substances produce the same appearances with Pettenkofer's test as do the biliary salts, it becomes necessary to apply the test in such a way as to exclude these sources of error. For this purpose the urine, about 50 cc., is evaporated to dryness over the water bath. The residue is extracted with strong alcohol, 5 cc.; the alcoholic solution is filtered and mixed with 50 cc. anhydrous ether. The ppt. formed is collected on a small filter, and, after having been washed with ether, is dissolved in 1 to 2 cc. H_2O. To the aqueous solution so obtained, Pettenkofer's test is applied as directed in § 56.

60. *Oliver's Peptone test.*—The reagent required is made by dissolving 2 gm. of pulverized peptone (Savory & Moore) and 0.27 gm. salicylic acid in 248 cc. of H_2O, and adding 2 cc. acetic acid. Filter till perfectly clear.

Dilute the urine to sp. gr. 1.008; pour some into a test-tube, and float upon its surface some of the reagent. An immediate cloudiness at the line of junction of the liquids indicates the presence of biliary salts.

Biliary Pigments.

61. Urine containing biliary pigments is always dark in color.

62. *Gmelin's test.*—Pour 3 cent. HNO_3 into a test-tube, add a piece of wood (1 cent. of the butt end of a match) and heat until the acid assumes a yellow color. Pour off the acid into another test-tube and cool it by immersing the tube in cold H_2O. When the acid is cold, float about 3 cent. of the urine to be tested upon its surface from a pipette. If biliary pigments be present, a green band is formed at the junction of the two liquids, which gradually rises higher and higher, and is succeeded from below by blue, reddish-violet, and yellow. The green color is much more distinctly marked than the others.

63. Shake the urine with ether. On standing, the ether separates as a *yellow* layer over the urine. Pour off the ether and float it on the surface of dilute bromine water in another test-tube. The ether gradually changes in color from yellow to blue.

64. *Paul's test.*—Add a few gtt. of a solution of methyl-violet to the urine. A ring of intense carmine color is formed on the surface. With normal urine a blue ring is formed.

The reaction is only produced with icteric urine, not with normal urine to which bile has been added.

QUANTITATIVE ANALYSIS OF URINE.

Reaction.

Alkalimetry and Acidimetry.

65. To determine the degree of acidity or alkalinity of the urine, solutions containing known quantities of oxalic acid and of caustic soda are required.

66. Weigh out 6.3 gms. of pure, crystallized oxalic acid $(C_2O_4H_2 + 2Aq = 126)$. Transfer it without loss to the measuring cylinder (Fig. 1, p. 3.); add H_2O to the 1,000 cc. mark, and agitate until solution is complete. The liquid so obtained is a *"Decinormal solution of oxalic acid,"* each cc. of which contains 0.0063 gm. of oxalic acid, equivalent to 0.004 gm. NaHO.

67. Weigh out 4.5 gm. of caustic soda. Dissolve in 60 cc. H_2O; add a lump of quicklime; boil about fifteen minutes; filter into the measuring cylinder; dilute to 900 cc. with H_2O, and mix.

Measure off 10 cc. of the decinormal oxalic acid solution with a pipette (Fig. 11); transfer it to a small beaker, and add to it 2 gtt. of an alcoholic solution of phenolphthaleïn (1 gm. in 100 cc.). Fill a burette (Fig. 12) with the soda solution to the 0 mark. Add the alkaline solution to the liquid in the beaker until the latter remains *faintly* red after stirring. Read the number of cc. of alkaline solution used from the graduation of the burette. This, multiplied by 100, gives the number of cc. of the solution containing 4.0 gms. of NaHO. Remove soda solution from the mixing cylinder until there remain exactly the number of cc. containing 4.0 gms. NaHO; add H_2O to the 1,000 cc. mark, and mix.

The solution so obtained is a "*Decinormal solution of caustic soda;*" each cc. of which contains 0.004 gm. NaHO,

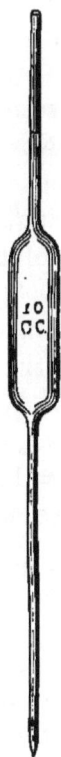
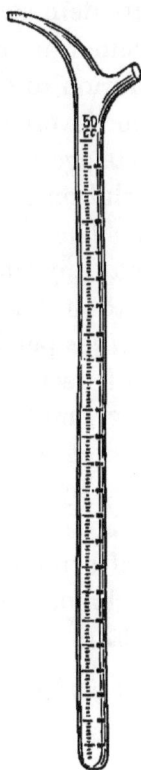
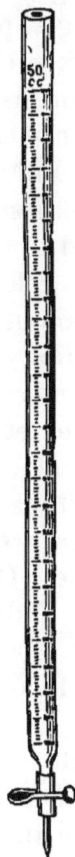

A.   B.

FIG. 11.   FIG. 12.

equivalent to 0.0063 $C_2O_4H_2 + 2$ Aq. The acid and alkaline solutions, therefore, neutralize each other, volume for volume.

The alkaline solution must be kept in glass-stoppered

bottles, the stoppers and necks of which have been coated with paraffin, and must be exposed to the air as little as possible.

68. To determine the degree of acidity in the urine, place two portions of 50 cc. each in two beakers, and add to each 4 gtt. phenolphthaleïn solution. Fill a burette to the 0 mark with the decinormal soda solution. Add portions of the alkaline solution to the contents of one of the beakers until a red color is produced, which persists on stirring. Fill the burette again to the 0 mark, and from it add 1 cc. less soda solution to the second beaker than was added to the first. The liquid in the second beaker should be yellow, without any tinge of red. Now continue the addition of soda solution to the second beaker, drop by drop, until a *faint red tinge* persists on stirring.

The number of cc. of decinormal soda solution used (the last burette reading), multiplied by 0.0063, gives the acidity of 50 cc. in grams of oxalic acid; from which the total acidity is determined by multiplying by the quantity of urine in twenty-four hours and dividing by 50.

Example. Quantity of urine in 24 hours = 1,350 cc.

Decinormal soda solution used = 14.6 cc.

14.6 × 0.0063 = 0.09198 = acidity of 50 cc. urine.

$$\frac{0.09198 \times 1350}{50} = 2.48 = \text{acidity of 24 hours in grams of}$$

oxalic acid.

69. To determine the degree of alkalinity, proceed as in § 68, using the decinormal oxalic acid solution in place of the soda solution in the burette; and adding the acid solution to the contents of the second beaker until the red color *just* disappears. The number of cc. of acid solution used, multiplied by 0.004, gives the alkalinity of 50 cc.; from which the total alkalinity is calculated as in § 68.

Example. Quantity of urine in 24 hours = 1,350 cc,

Decinormal oxalic acid solution used $= 7.4$ cc.

$7.4 \times 0.004 = 0.0296 =$ alkalinity of 50 cc. urine.

$\dfrac{0.0296 \times 1,350}{50} = 0.80 =$ alkalinity of 24 hours in grams of caustic soda.

70. The normal acidity of twenty-four hours of the urine is equal to two to four grams of oxalic acid.

Chlorides.

71. The solutions required are: 1. *A standard solution of silver nitrate*, made by dissolving 29.075 gms. of pure, fused, and recrystallized $AgNO_3$ in 1,000 cc. H_2O. This solution must be kept in bottles of amber glass. 2. *A solution of neutral potassium chromate;* 10 gms. to 100 cc. H_2O.

72. To conduct the determination, 5 cc. of urine are placed in a platinum basin, 2 gms. of $NaNO_3$ (free from chloride) are added. The whole is evaporated to dryness over the water bath, and the residue gradually heated until a colorless fused mass remains. This residue, after cooling, is dissolved in H_2O, the soln. transferred to a small beaker, treated with pure, dil. HNO_3 to faintly acid reaction, and neutralized with powdered $CaCO_3$; 2 gtt. of the chromate soln. are now added, and finally the silver soln. from a burette (previously filled with $AgNO_3$ soln. to the 0 mark), during constant stirring of the contents of the beaker, until a faint reddish tinge remains permanent. Each cc. of the $AgNO_3$ soln. used represents 0.01 gm. $NaCl$ (or 0.0607 gms. Cl) in 5 cc. urine; from which the $NaCl$ in twenty-four hours is calculated.

Example. Urine in 24 hours $= 1,260$ cc.

Silver soln. used $= 6.7$ cc.

$\dfrac{0.01 \times 6.7}{5} \times 1,260 = 16.88$ gms. $NaCl$ in 24 hours.

N. B.—This process cannot be used during administration of bromides or iodides.

73. The amount of Cl voided by a normal male adult, upon normal diet, is about 10 grams in twenty-four hours, equivalent to 16.5 gms. NaCl.

Phosphates.

74. The solutions required are: 1. *A standard solution of disodic phosphate,* made by dissolving 10.085 gms. of crystallized, non-effloresced disodic phosphate ($Na_2HPO_4 + 12$ Aq.) in H_2O, and diluting the solution to 1 litre. Fifty cc. of this soln. contain 0.1 gm. phosphoric anhydride P_2O_5. 2. *An acid solution of sodium acetate,* made by dissolving 100 gms. $NaC_2H_3O_2 + 3$ Aq. in 100 cc. H_2O, adding 100 cc. glacial $HC_2H_3O_2$, and diluting with H_2O to 1,000 cc. 3. *A solution of potassium ferrocyanide;* 10 gms. in 100 cc. H_2O. 4. *A standard solution of uranic acetate.* To obtain this soln., a soln. of approximate strength is first made by dissolving 33 gms. of yellow uranic oxide in glacial acetic acid, and diluting with H_2O to 900 cc. in the mixing cylinder. Solution No. 1 serves to determine the true strength of this soln., as follows: 50 cc. of soln. 1 are placed in a beaker, and 5 cc. of soln. 2 are added. The mixture is heated on the water bath, and the uranium soln. gradually added from a burette until a drop of the liquid, taken from the beaker on a stirring-rod, produces a brown color when brought in contact with a drop of soln. 3. At this point, the reading of the burette, which indicates the number of cc. of the uranium soln., corresponding to 0.1 gm. P_2O_5, is taken. This reading, multiplied by 50, gives the number of cc. uranium soln. equivalent to 5 gms. P_2O_5. Remove uranium soln. from the mixing cylinder until there remain the number of cc. which have been found to be equivalent to 5 gm. P_2O_5; add H_2O to the 1,000 cc.

mark, and mix. The uranium solution so standardized is of such strength that each cc. is equivalent to 0.005 gm. P_2O_5.

75. To determine the *total phosphoric anhydride* in the urine: 50 cc. are placed in a beaker, 5 cc. sodium acetate soln. are added, and the mixture heated on the water bath. When warm, the standard uranium soln. is added from a burette until a drop, removed from the beaker with a stirring-rod, produces a faint brown tinge when brought in contact with a drop of ferrocyanide soln. The burette reading taken at this point and multiplied by 0.005 gives the amount of P_2O_5 in 50 cc. urine; and this, multiplied by $\frac{1}{50}$ the amount of urine eliminated in twenty-four hours, gives the daily elimination in grams of P_2O_5.

Example. Urine in 24 hours = 1,180 cc.
Uranium solution used = 24.3 cc.
$24.3 \times .005 = 0.1215.$

$$\frac{1,180 \times 0.1215}{50} = 2.87 = \text{grams } P_2O_5 \text{ in 24 hours.}$$

76. To determine the *phosphoric anhydride corresponding to earthy phosphates*, 100 cc. of the urine are rendered alkaline with NH_4HO.and set aside for twelve hours. Collect the ppt. on a filter, wash it with dilute ammonium hydrate soln. (1 : 3). Perforate the point of the filter, and wash the ppt. into a small beaker; dissolve in as little acetic acid as possible; make up the solution to about 50 cc. with H_2O, add 5 cc. sodium acetate soln., and titrate as in § 75.

N. B.—In standardizing (§ 74) the uranium soln., and in using it (§ 75, § 76), time will be saved by taking two quantities of 50 cc. each of the phosphate soln. or urine. Make an approximate determination with one beaker, by adding to it 15 cc. of the uranium soln., and then further quantities of 2 cc. each until the red color is obtained with ferrocyanide. Then add to the second beaker an amount of uranium soln. equal to that which last failed to respond to the ferrocyanide soln. in the first sample, and continue the addition of uranium soln., drop by drop, until the final reaction is obtained.

77. The normal amount of phosphoric anhydride in twenty-four hours is 2.5 to 3.5 grams, of which 0.8 to 1.2 grams are in combination as earthy phosphates, and 1.7 to 2.3 as alkaline phosphates.

Sulphates.

78. To 100 cc. of the urine add 5 cc. HCl; heat to near boiling; add $BaCl_2$ soln. in slight excess; let the beaker containing the mixture stand on the water bath until the ppt. has subsided; decant the clear liquid through a small filter without disturbing the ppt.; add hot water to the beaker; let the ppt. settle again, decant as before, and continue this washing by decantation until a portion of the filtrate no longer becomes cloudy on addition of dil. H_2SO_4. Transfer the ppt. to the filter by the aid of the wash bottle (Fig. 7, p. 10), and dry in the water oven. Burn the filter in a weighed platinum crucible until white. Weigh the crucible, ash, and $BaSO_4$, and from this weight subtract that of the crucible and filter ash. The difference, multiplied by 0.421, is the weight of sulphuric acid, H_2SO_4 in 100 cc. urine; and this, multiplied by $\frac{1}{100}$ of the quantity in twenty-four hours, is the amount of H_2SO_4 eliminated in twenty-four hours.

Example. Quantity of urine in 24 hours = 1,320 cc.

Weight of platinum crucible, filter-ash, and $BaSO_4$ =17.8932

"   "   "   "   and filter-ash   =17.4863

Weight of $BaSO_4$ = 0.4069

$0.4069 \times 0.421 = 0.1713 =$ grams H_2SO_4 in 100 cc.

0.1713 × 13.20 = 2.26 = grams H_2SO_4 in 24 hours.

79. The normal daily elimination of H_2SO_4 is from 2 to 2.5 grams.

Urea.

80. Urine containing an excess of urea has a high specific gravity, while that which is deficient in urea is of lower specific gravity than normal.

81. Take two watch glasses. Into one put 5 gtt. of the urine, into the other 10 gtt. Evaporate the latter over the water bath until it has been reduced to the volume of the

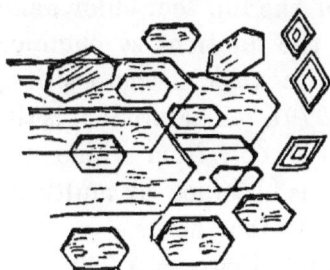

former. Cool the contents of both watch glasses to about 15° and add to each 3 gtt. of cold, colorless, concentrated HNO_3. If, after a few moments, crystals of urea nitrate appear in both watch glasses, the urine contains an excess of urea; if crystals do not form in either watch glass, the

FIG. 13.

proportion of urea is deficient; while if crystals appear in one and not in the other, the amount of urea is about normal.

This method is only capable of showing roughly an increase or a diminution in the proportion of urea. Two precautions are to be observed in its use: 1. The *amorphous* deposit produced in albuminous urine is not to be mistaken for the *crystalline* urea nitrate. 2. The process can be applied as described above only when the quantity of urine in twenty-four hours is about normal. If it be greater or less than normal, a modification is necessary. If, for instance, the quantity of urine in twenty-four hours be half the normal, two samples of 5 gtt. each are to be taken, one of which is to be diluted with 5 gtt. H_2O. If the quantity in twenty-four hours be double the normal, two samples are to be taken, one of 10 gtt., the other of 20 gtt., and both reduced to 5 gtt. by evaporation.

82. *Fowler's method.*—Determine the sp. gr. of the urine and the sp. gr. of some liq. sodæ chlorinatæ (Squibb) at the same temperature. Mix one volume of the urine with seven volumes of the liq. sod. chlor. After the violence of the reaction has subsided, shake the mixture from time to time during an hour. Determine the sp. gr. of the mixture at the same temperature at which the former observations were made. Add once the sp. gr. of the urine to seven times the sp. gr. of the liq. sod. chlor., and divide the sum by eight. From the quotient so obtained subtract the sp. gr. of the mixture after decomposition, and multiply the difference by 0.7791. The product is the amount of urea in grams in 100 cc.; from which the elimination in twenty-four hours is obtained by multiplying by $\frac{1}{100}$ of the quantity in twenty-four hours.

Example. Quantity of urine in 24 hours = 1,240 cc.

Specific gravity of liq. sod. chlor. = 1,042
"   "   " urine   = 1,020
"   "   " mixture   = 1,036.2

$$\frac{1,042 \times 7 + 1,020}{8} = 1,039.25.\ 1,039.3 - 1,036.2 = 3.1$$

$0.7791 \times 3.1 \times 12.40 = 29.95 =$ grams of urea in 24 hours.

83. For accurate determinations of the quantity of urea, one of the modifications of the Knop-Hüfner process is recommended (see "Manual," p. 193, and Charles' "Physiological Chem.," pp. 350 et seq.).

Uric Acid.

84. Acidulate 200 cc. of the filtered urine with 10 cc. HCl, and set it aside in a cool place for forty-eight hours.

Wash a small filter with dil. HCl, dry it, inclose it between two watch-glasses, held together by a brass clamp, and de. termine the weight of the whole. Collect the crystals which have formed in the acidulated urine upon the weighed filter, detaching such crystals as adhere to the wall of the vessel by rubbing with a small section of rubber tubing, slipped over the end of a glass rod, and washing the deposit on to the filter with portions of the filtrate. When the ppt. is all on the filter wash it by the successive addition of small portions of H_2O, until the filtrate is no longer acid. The filter and contents are now dried, inclosed between the watch-glasses, and weighed. This last weight, minus that first determined, is the weight of uric acid in 200 cc. urine; and this, multiplied by $\frac{1}{200}$ the amount of urine in twenty-four hours, is the amount in twenty-four hours.

The amount of wash water used should not exceed 35 cc. If more should be used, add 0.043 mgm. to the weight of uric acid in 200 cc. urine for every extra cc. of wash water.

Example. Urine in 24 hours = 1,230 cc.

Weight of watch-glasses, clamp, filter, and uric acid	36.3275
Weight of watch-glasses, clamp, and filter	36.1948

Uric acid in 200 cc.	0.1327
Correction for wash water	0.0004

45 cc. wash water used . ·. .043 × 10 = 0.43 mgm.

Uric acid in 200 cc. corrected 0.1331

$$\frac{0.1331 \times 1,230}{200} = 0.8185 = \text{grams uric acid in 24 hours.}$$

85. The normal elimination of uric acid in twenty-four hours is from 0.5 to 1.0 gram.

Albumin.

86. *Esbach's method.*—For this method a tube 1.5 cent. in diameter and 15 cent. long, graduated into grams, and having two marks, one near the middle, the other near the top, is required; also a reagent made by adding 50 cc. acetic acid to 950 cc. of a solution of picric acid containing 10 gms. to the L.

If the urine be alkaline, render it acid with acetic acid. If the urine be of less sp. gr. than 1.008, fill the tube to the lower mark with it; add the reagent to the upper mark; close the opening of the tube with the finger and turn it upside down several times. The tube is now allowed to remain at rest twelve hours, after which time the amount of albumin is read off on the graduation.

If the sp. gr. of the urine be above 1.008, it is to be diluted with water, the degree of dilution being considered in the final result.

Results roughly approximate.

87. *Gravimetric method.*—Place 100 cc. of the clear urine in a beaker of 200 cc. capacity; if alkaline, acidulate with acetic acid. Heat the beaker over the water-bath, add 1–2 gtt. acetic acid, and heat to boiling; continue boiling gently until the diffuse ppt. has collected in lumps. Have ready a small filter whose weight, with that of watch-glasses and clamp (see § 84), has been determined; collect the coagulated albumin upon the filter, wash with H_2O containing a little NH_4HO, then with boiling H_2O until the filtrate no longer forms a ppt. with $AgNO_3$, then with alcohol, and finally with ether. Dry the filter and contents in the air oven, and weigh between the watch-glasses. The difference between this last weight and the one first determined is the weight of dry albumin in 100 cc. urine, which, multiplied by $\frac{1}{100}$ the quantity in twenty-four hours, gives the elimination of albumin in twenty-four hours.

If the urine be highly albuminous, it is best to operate upon 20 or 50 cc., diluted with 80 or 50 cc. H_2O, and multiply to obtain the final result by $\frac{1}{20}$ or $\frac{1}{50}$ the amount of urine in twenty-four hours.

Glucose.

88. *Fehling's method.*—The solution is made as follows:

I. Dissolve cupric sulphate   51.98 grams,
     in water to   500.00 cc.
II. Dissolve Rochelle salt   259.9 grams,
    in sodium hydrate soln. sp. gr. 1.12 to 1,000 cc.

When required for use, one volume of I. is to be mixed with two volumes of II. The copper contained in 10 cc. of this mixture is precipitated completely, as cuprous oxide, by 0.05 gram of glucose.

89. To determine the quantity of sugar, place 10 cc. of the mixed soln. in a flask of about 250 cc. capacity; dilute with H_2O to about 30 cc. and heat to boiling. On the other hand, the urine to be tested is diluted, and thoroughly mixed with four volumes of H_2O if it be poor in sugar, or with nine volumes of H_2O if highly saccharine, and a burette filled with the mixture. When the Fehling soln. boils, add a few gtt. NH_4HO and then 5 cc. of the urine from the burette, boil again, and continue the alternate addition of diluted urine and boiling of the mixture until the blue color is quite faint. Now add the diluted urine in quantities of 1 cc. at a time, boiling after each addition until the blue color just disappears. Have ready a small filter and, having filtered through it a few gtt. of the hot mixture, accidulate the filtrate with acetic acid, and add to it 1 gtt. soln. of potassium ferrocyanide. If a brownish tinge be produced, add another $\frac{1}{2}$ cc. of dil. urine to the flask, boil and test with ferrocyanide as before. Continue this proceeding until no brown tinge is produced. The burette reading, taken at this point, gives the number of cc. of dilute urine containing 0.05 gm. glucose, and this, divided by 5 or 10, according as the urine was diluted with 4 or 9 volumes of H_2O, gives the number of cc. of urine containg 0.05 gm. sugar. The number of cc. urine passed in twenty-four hours, divided by 20 times the number of cc. containing 0.05 gm. glucose, gives the elimination of glucose in twenty-four hours in grams.

Example. Urine in 24 hours = 2,436 cc.

Fehling's soln. used = 10 cc.

Urine diluted with 4 vols. H_2O

Burette reading = 18.5 cc.

$$\frac{18.5}{5} = 3.7 = \text{cc. urine containing } 0.05 \text{ gm. glucose.}$$

$$\frac{2,436}{3.7 \times 20} = 32.92 = \text{grams glucose eliminated in 24 hours.}$$

URINARY DEPOSITS.

90. Shake the urine to be examined, fill a conical glass (Fig. 14) with it, cover the glass with a watch-glass or glass plate, and set it aside until any solid particles have subsided to the bottom.

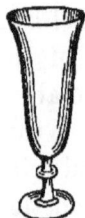

Crystalline deposits settle in a few hours, but if the urine have been found to contain albumin, and casts are consequently to be looked for, twelve hours must be allowed to elapse to insure complete deposition.

Fig. 14.

After the deposit has collected at the point of the glass, some of the sediment is removed with a pipette. Hold the pipette in such a manner that its upper opening is closed by the forefinger, and bring the point down into the layer of sediment, free the upper opening for an instant, close it again, and withdraw the pipette. Transfer a small quantity of urine and sediment from the pipette to a glass slide, upon which a ring of cement has been made and allowed to dry, put on a clean cover glass, remove the excess of liquid from the slide with bibulous paper and examine with the microscope.

Unorganized Deposits.

91. URIC ACID.—Deposits of uric acid occur in acid urines; are always crystalline, of the forms shown in Fig. 15, of which *b* are exceptional forms, and *a* of common

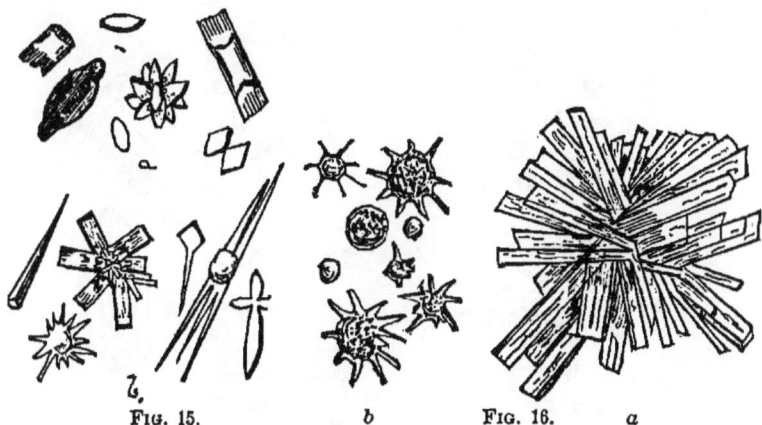

FIG. 15.   *b*   FIG. 16.   *a*

occurrence; almost invariably of a color varying from light yellow to dark red or brown. Frequently they are of sufficient size to be visible to the unaided eye. Deposits of uric acid respond to the murexid test, § 24, and dissolve when warmed with NaHO soln.

92. AMORPHOUS, ACID URATES consist principally of acid sodium urate, accompanied sometimes with much smaller quantities of the potassium, calcium, and ammonium salts. The deposit is amorphous, composed of minute granular particles, sometimes colorless, but frequently yellow or red ("brick dust" or "lateritious" sediment), produced in acid urine. Urine cloudy from the presence of amorphous urates becomes clear when heated.

93. CRYSTALLINE URATES. —*Acid sodium urate* sometimes crystallizes from the urine undergoing acid or incipient alkaline fermentation, in the form of prisms arranged in stellate bundles (Fig. 16, *a*). Later in the fermentative process, when ammonia is produced, the highly colored spherical crystals, with or without spines (Fig. 16, *b*), of acid ammonium urate are produced.

94. CALCIUM OXALATE is observed sometimes in acid urine, accompanying crystals of uric acid, sometimes in

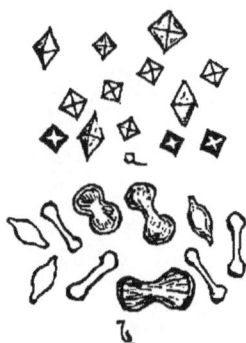

FIG. 17.

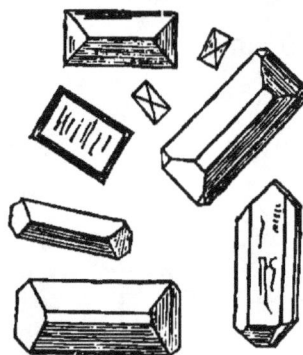

FIG. 18.

alkaline or neutral urine, along with crystals of triple phosphate. These crystals are usually very minute octahedra (Fig. 17, *a*), and occasionally in "dumb-bell" forms (Fig. 17, *b*).

95. AMMONIO-MAGNESIAN PHOSPHATE—*triple phosphate*—occurs in slightly acid or alkaline urine, particularly of the shapes shown in Fig. 18, sufficiently large to be visible as shining specks when the vessel containing the urine is rotated in sunlight. Occasionally it forms stars shaped groups of feathery crystals.

96. CALCIUM PHOSPHATE is deposited under the same

conditions as ammonio-magnesian phosphate. The deposit is usually amorphous, and increases on the application of heat, but disappears on the addition of a mineral acid. Occasionally calcium phosphate crystallizes from the urine, either in wedge-shaped crystals, arranged in rosettes, their points uniting (Fig. 19), or in spherical crystals, or, more rarely, in dumb-bells.

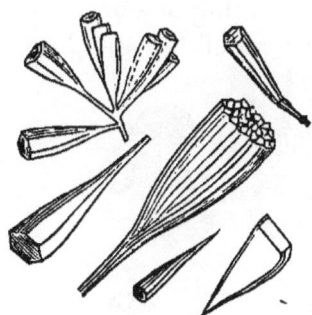

FIG. 19.

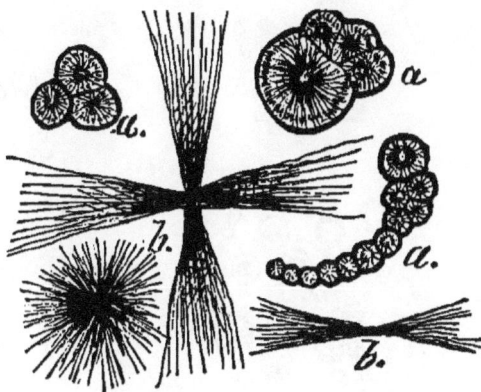

FIG. 20.

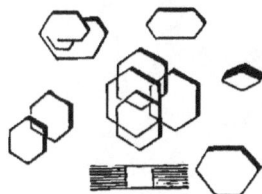

FIG. 21.

97. LEUCIN AND TYROSIN always occur together, and are found only in urines containing biliary pigments. The former substance forms yellow, highly refracting spheres of varying size, marked with radiating and concentric striations (Fig. 20, *a*). Tyrosin crystallizes in bundles of delicate hair-like crystals, arranged in brush-like groups (Fig. 20, *b*).

98. CYSTIN is of rare occurrence. It appears as a yellowish deposit in pale, acid, or alkaline urine; which, when examined microscopically, is found to consist of hexagonal plates, either colorless or pigmented (Fig. 21). It dissolves in NH_4HO and crystallizes out again an evaporation of the solution.

Organized Deposits.

99. MUCUS OR PUS CORPUSCLES are rounded, granular cells, larger than blood-corpuscles, containing one or more nuclei (Fig. 22). Water causes them to swell up and lose

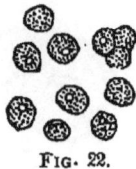

FIG. 22.

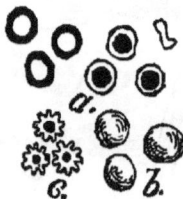

FIG. 24.

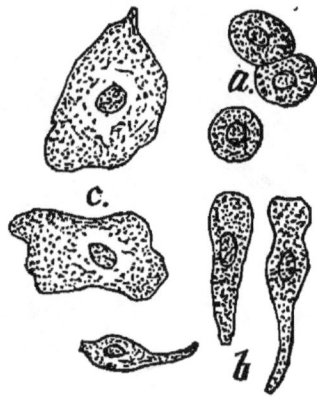

FIG. 23.

their granular marking; the nuclei become more distinct, and the body of the cell gradually becomes invisible. Dilute acetic acid (20%) produces the same changes more rapidly.

100. EPITHELIUM.—The epithelial cells met with in urine are: 1. *Round epithelial cells*, from the convoluted tubes, the pelvis of the kidney, the bladder, and the male urethra; are rounded granular bodies, larger than pus-corpuscles, containing a single nucleus (Fig. 23, *a*). 2. *Columnar or conical epithelial cells*, from the pelvis of the kidney, the ureters and urethra, are elongated, conical bodies, granular, and containing a single nucleus near the middle (Fig. 23, *b*). 3. *Flat epithelial cells*, from the bladder and vagina, are large, irregular, scale-like bodies, faintly granular, and containing a single nucleus (Fig. 23, *c*).

100. BLOOD-CORPUSCLES appear in urine as rounded bodies, whose centres and peripheries alternate in light and shadow as the objective is moved toward or away from the slide (Fig. 24, *a*). If the urine be dilute, the blood-discs

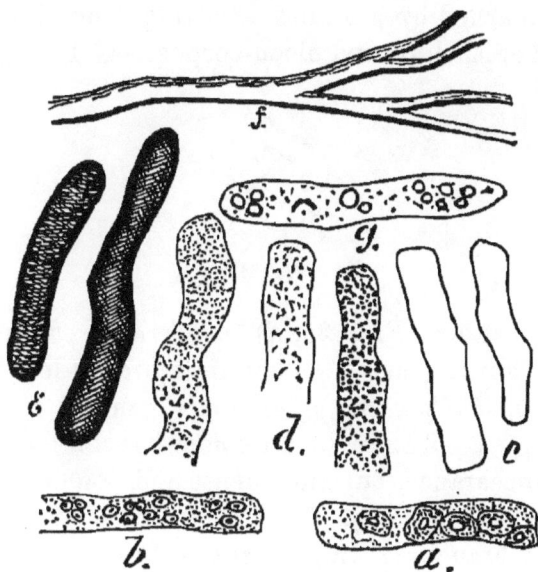

FIG. 25.

lose their concavity, swell up, and no longer show alternations of light and shadow (Fig. 24, *b*); finally they become invisible. If the urine be concentrated, their concavity becomes greater, they shrink, and finally assume a crenated form (Fig. 24, *c*).

101. CASTS are moulds of the uriniferous tubules, of which the following varieties occur: 1. *Epithelial casts* are clear, cylindrical bodies, in whose surfaces epithelium from the tubules is imbedded (Fig. 25, *a*). 2. *Blood casts* are casts marked with granules and having blood-corpuscles imbedded in them (Fig. 25, *b*). 3. *Hyaline casts* are perfectly clear, transparent cylinders, without any markings (Fig. 25, *c*) which, being of about the same index of refracsion as the urine, may be readily overlooked if the examination be not very carefully made. Their detection is facilitated by adding a drop of a solution of fuchsin to the deposit before putting on the cover glass. 4. *Granular casts* are marked by granules resulting from the disintegration of epithelium and blood-corpuscles. They are either

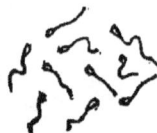

Fig. 26.

highly granular (Fig. 25, *d*), *moderately granular*, or *faintly granular*, as they contain more or less granular matter. 5. *Fatty casts*, *or oil casts*, contain oil globules (Fig. 25, *g*). 6. *Waxy casts* are somewhat similar to hyaline casts in appearance, but more dense and somewhat resembling wax (Fig. 25, *e*). 7. *Mucous casts* are very long, frequently branching, transparent bodies (Fig. 25, *f*).

102. SPERMATOZOA are minute, tadpole-like bodies (Fig. 26), which, when present in urine, do not exhibit the vibrating motion with which they are endowed during life.

QUALITATIVE ANALYSIS OF URINARY CALCULI.

103. If the calculus be large, and if it is to be preserved, saw it in two with a hack-saw and use the saw-dust for analysis, keeping that portion of the dust which is produced while sawing through the centre of the stone separate from the other. If the calculus be small, break it; separate the nucleus, if there be one, powder the nucleus and a portion of the body of the stone separately, and make an independent analysis of each.

104. In using the following scheme, take a separate portion of the powder for each operation unless otherwise directed.

SCHEME OF ANALYSIS.

1. Heat on platinum foil until colorless:
   - *a.* It is entirely volatile 2
   - *b.* A residue remains........................... 5

2. Moisten with HNO_3; evaporate to dryness over the water bath; add NH_4HO:
   - *a.* A red color is produced.................... 3
   - *b.* No red color is produced.................. 4

3. Treat with KHO, without heating:
   - *a.* An ammoniacal odor is produced,

     Ammonium urate.

   - *b.* No ammoniacal odor is produced... *Uric acid.*

4. *a.* The HNO_3 soln. becomes yellow when evaporated; the yellow residue becomes reddish-yellow on addition of KHO, and on heating with KHO, violet red,

   Xanthin.

b. The HNO$_3$ soln. becomes dark brown on evaporation............................. *Cystin.*

5. Moisten with HNO$_3$, evaporate to dryness over the water bath; add NH$_4$HO:
    a. A red color is produced.................. 6
    b. No red color is produced............... 9

6. Heat before the blow-pipe on platinum foil:
    a. Fuses...... 7
    b. Does not fuse......................... 8

7. Bring into blue flame on clean platinum wire:
    a. Flame colored yellow.......... *Sodium urate.*
    b. Flame violet when observed through blue glass,
                  Potassium urate.

8. The residue from 6:
    a. Dissolves in dil. HCl with effervescence; the soln. forms a white ppt. with ammonium oxalate,
                   Calcium urate.
    b. Dissolves with slight effervescence in dil. H$_2$SO$_4$; the soln. neutralized with NH$_4$HO gives a white ppt. with Na$_2$HPO$_4$............... .... *Magnesium urate.*

9. Heat on platinum foil:
    a. It fuses:..... *Ammonio-magnesian phosphate.*
    b. It does not fuse.......................10

10. The residue from 9, moistened with H$_2$O, and tested with red litmus paper, is:
    a. Alkaline.............................11
    b. Not alkaline............ *Tricalcic phosphate.*

11. The original substance dissolves in HCl:
    a. With effervescence........ *Calcium carbonate.*
    b. Without effervescence....... *Calcium oxalate.*

DETECTION OF POISONS.

105. The identification of any of the accessible poisons when unmixed with other substances does not present any serious difficulty. When, however, the poison is mixed with a large proportion of foreign substances, as in an article of food, in the contents of the stomach or in the viscera, the reactions upon which we depend are masked or modified to such a degree that no reliance is to be placed upon them. Consequently, in searching for a poison in organic mixtures the first step, preliminary to the actual testing, is the separation of the poison from other substances in a condition as pure as possible, and with as little loss as may be.

106. Analytically, poisons are divided into three classes, according to the methods used in their separation from organic mixtures: 1. Volatile Poisons. 2. Mineral Poisons. 3. Organic Poisons.

VOLATILE POISONS.

107. Those poisons which may be separated from the materials under examination by the process of distillation are included in this class. The most important are: Phosphorus, Hydrocyanic Acid, Alcohol, Ether, Chloroform, Chloral, Benzol and its derivatives, including Carbolic Acid.

108. To separate poisons of this class, the contents of the stomach (or other substance to be examined), diluted with H_2O if necessary, are slightly acidulated with dilute H_2SO_4 and placed in a flask, which should be only half

filled; the flask is then connected with a Liebig's condenser and heated over a sand bath. The distillation is continued until two-thirds of the liquid have distilled over,
and the distillate is collected in three separate portions.
The distillates are then to be tested for individual poisons
by suitable reagents.

Phosphorus. P.

109. The material gives off an odor of garlic, and (alcohol, ether, and oil of turpentine being absent) is luminous when shaken in the dark.

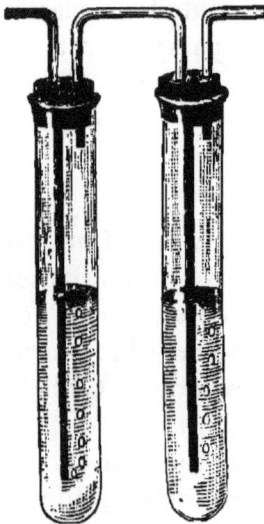

Fig. 27.

110. It is advisable in cases of
suspected phosphorus poisoning to
spread the suspected material out
on a clean plate, and examine it
in a dark room for any luminous
points. It must not be forgotten,
however, that muscular and other
animal tissues may be phosphores-
cent in absence of phosphorus.

111. If the presence of phosphorus be suspected, the process,
§ 108, is to be somewhat modified.
It is to be conducted in a dark
room with a screen interposed between the condenser and the source
of heat. If no luminous ring (§
112) be observed when one-third
of the liquid has distilled over, remove the condenser and
substitute for it the apparatus shown in Fig. 27, charged
with $AgNO_3$ soln., and continue the distillation while a
current of CO_2 is passed through the entire apparatus.
If phosphorus be present, the $AgNO_3$ soln. blackens. If
this occur, collect the black deposit formed and introduce

it into an apparatus in which hydrogen is generated, and ignite the escaping gas at a platinum jet. In the presence of phosphorus, a bright green core appears in the flame.

112. During the distillation, § 111, a luminous band is observed at the point of greatest condensation in the condenser. If, however, the liquid in the flask contains alcohol or ether, this luminous band does not appear until after one-third of the liquid has been distilled. If oil of turpentine be present, the luminous band does not appear at all.

113. Examine the distillate for globules of P, which are recognized by their yellow, waxy appearance, their odor, their luminosity in the dark, and the bluing of paper moistened with iodide of potassium and starch when exposed to the vapors which they give off.

114. ANTIDOTES.—No chemical antidote known. Remove unabsorbed poison with stomach-pump, $ZnSO_4$ or apomorphia. Old French oil of turpentine. Prohibit fats and oils, which favor absorption.

Hydrocyanic Acid--Prussic Acid (HCN).

115. Note the odor of bitter almonds, or peach blossoms

116. Add $AgNO_3$ to the soln.; a dense white ppt. Collect the ppt. on a filter, and warm a part with HNO_3; the ppt. dissolves. Treat remainder of ppt. with KCN soln.; it dissolves.

117. Add NH_4HS to soln. and evaporate to dryness on water-bath; add Fe_2Cl_6 to residue; a deep red color.

118. Add KHO, and then an old soln. of $FeSO_4$; a greenish ppt. Add HCl; the ppt. dissolves partly, forming a deep blue soln.

119. Add dil. soln. of picric acid, heat, and allow to cool; a deep red color.

120. Moisten a piece of filter paper with a freshly prepared alcoholic soln. of guaiacum; dip the paper into a very dilute soln. $CuSO_4$, and hold it over a vessel from which vapor of HCN is given off; the paper turns bright blue.

121. ANTIDOTES.—A mixture of ferrous and ferric sulphates dissolved in H_2O and alkalinized with KHO is a chemical antidote. The action of the poison is usually so rapid, however, that it is of little service. Stomach pump, cold affusion, artificial respiration, galvanism, inhalation of ammonia, of chlorine (?). Atropine hypodermically (?).

Alcohol. C_2H_5HO.

122. Heat with a small quantity of a cooled mixture of H_2SO_4 and aqueous soln. of potassium dichromate; the liquid turns green, and the peculiar odor of aldehyde is given off.

123. Dissolve in the liquid a small quantity of iodine, add KHO soln. guttatim until the liquid is just decolorized, and warm; a yellowish crystalline ppt. immediately or after a time, and the odor of iodoform.

124. Add HNO_3 and warm; odor of nitrous ether. Add soln. mercurous nitrate with excess HNO_3 and heat; a yellow-gray ppt. Collect ppt., wash, and dry; explodes when struck with hammer.

125. Mix slowly with an equal volume H_2SO_4; add some powdered sodium acetate, and heat; odor of acetic ether.

Chloroform. $CHCl_3$.

126. Add a few gtt. aniline to 3 cc. alcoholic soln. of KHO, and then 2 cc. of the liquid to be tested, and heat. In the presence of chloroform, an intense, disagreeable, and characteristic odor, due to the formation of isobenzonitril, is produced.

127. Dissolve about 0.01 gm. of β naphthol in a small quantity of KHO soln., warm, and add the suspected liquid: a blue color is produced.

128. Place the liquid to be examined, which should be faintly acidulated with H_2SO_4 if not already acid. in a flask. Fit the flask with a cork through which pass two right-angled tubes, one of which dips to near the bottom of the flask. Connect this longer tube with a bellows or gasometer, from which a slow current of air is made to pass through the apparatus during the process. The shorter tube is connected with about a foot of Bohemian tubing, whose other end communicates with a right-angled tube dipping into a solution of $AgNO_3$, or with a bulb apparatus filled with $AgNO_3$ soln. Heat the flask over a water-bath, and heat about six inches of the Bohemian tube to bright redness. In the presence of $CHCl_3$ a white ppt. of AgCl, soluble in NH_4HO, insoluble in HNO_3, is formed in the $AgNO_3$ soln.

129. ANTIDOTES.—No chemical antidote is known. Cold douche, galvanism, fresh air, artificial respiration, inhalation of ammonia.

Chloral—Trichloraldehyde. C_2HCl_3O.

130. The substance to be examined is first treated as in § 128. If no ppt. be produced in the $AgNO_3$ soln., the liquid in the flask is rendered *alkaline* with KHO soln., and the process continued. If now a ppt. be formed in the $AgNO_3$ soln., the flask is connected with a condenser and more strongly heated. Portions of the distillate are then tested according to §§ 126, 127 for chloroform, resulting from the decomposition of the chloral by the alkali.

131. ANTIDOTES.—No chemical antidote. Stomach-pump, tea, coffee, galvanism, artificial respiration, cold douche, ammonia by inhalation.

Phenol—Carbolic Acid. C_6H_6HO.

132. Odor of carbolic acid.

133. Mix with one-quarter volume NH_4HO; add 1–2 gtt. sodium hypochlorite soln. and warm: a blue or green color. Add HCl to acid reaction: turns red.

134. Add 1–2 gtt. of the liquid to a little HCl, mix; add 1 gtt. HNO_3: a purple-red color.

135. Boil with HNO_3 as long as red fumes are given off. Neutralize with KHO: a yellow, crystalline ppt.

136. Add a few gtt. $FeSO_4$ soln.: a lilac color.

137. Float liquid to be tested on H_2SO_4; add powdered KNO_3: violet color.

138. Add excess of bromine water: a yellowish-white ppt.

139. ANTIDOTES.—Emetics, white of egg, stimulants.

MINERAL POISONS.

MINERAL ACIDS AND ALKALIES.

140. These substances are corrosives rather than true poisons, as their deleterious effects are produced by destruction of or injury to important viscera with which they come into immediate contact, while the true poisons act only after absorption into the circulation.

141. The presence of strong acids or alkalies in the stomach is indicated by corrosion or even perforation of the viscus, and by a strongly acid or alkaline reaction of the contents. It must not be forgotten that the contents of the stomach may have been rendered alkaline after the ingestion of acids, or acid after alkalies have been taken, by the administration of antidotes.

142. In all cases of corrosion by mineral acids or alkalies (except nitric acid) a quantitative analysis should be made, and the amount found compared with that normally present, as sulphates, chlorides, and salts of sodium and potassium are normal constituents of body.

Sulphuric Acid. H_2SO_4.

143. With $BaCl_2$ a copious, white ppt., insoluble in HCl. This reaction does not prove the presence of *free* sulphuric acid, as it is also observed with soluble sulphates.

144. Add powdered lead chromate, boil, filter; add KI and carbon bisulphide, and agitate. The CS_2 is colored violet. Agitate another portion of the liquid with CS_2 after addition of KI: no violet color should be produced.

145. Dissolve 3 per cent of cane-sugar in the liquid, moisten a piece of filter paper with it and dry: the paper turns brown or black.

146. Moisten a little veratria with the liquid, and evaporate over the water-bath to dryness: a crimson color.

Hydrochloric Acid. HCl.

147. Add $AgNO_3$: a white ppt soluble in NH_4HO, insoluble in HNO_3. Observed also with chlorides.

148. Add mercurous nitrate: a white ppt., which turns black on addition of NH_4HO. Observed also with chlorides.

149. Heat the liquid with powdered black oxide of manganese (MnO_2): chlorine is given off; recognizable by its odor, its yellow color, and by its power of turning paper containing starch and potassium iodide blue.

Nitric Acid. HNO₃.

150. Float upon the liquid a soln. of ferrous sulphate: a brown band appears at the junction of the liquids. A nitrate only responds to this test after addition of H_2SO_4.

151. Moisten a crystal of brucine with the liquid: a bright carmine-red color. Nitrates respond to this test after addition of H_2SO_4.

152. Dissolve 252 pts. of cyanide of mercury and 266 pts. KI in H_2O, evaporate to crystallization; separate, and dry the crystals. A crystal introduced into nitric acid turns black.

153. Acidulate the (colorless) liquid with HCl, and add 1-2 gtt. indigo-carmine soln.: the blue color is discharged.

154. ANTIDOTES FOR MINERAL ACIDS.—Magnesia usta, suspended in water, or, failing this, soap. Neither the carbonates of the alkalies, chalk, or carbonate of magnesia should be used, as the gas liberated from them may cause serious distention of the weakened walls of the stomach. The stomach-pump should *never* be used. It will frequently be necessary to sustain life by nutritive enemata. Opium to allay pain.

Caustic Potassa—Potassium Hydrate. KHO.

155. Add HCl and then $PtCl_4$ soln.: a yellow crystalline ppt. A similar ppt. is obtained with ammonium chloride.

156. Concentrate the soln., render it neutral with Na_2CO_3 if acid, and add concentrated soln. of tartaric acid: a white ppt. A similar ppt. with ammonium salts.

157. Add soln. of hydrofluosilicic acid : a white, gelatinous ppt., insoluble in HCl. A similar ppt. with sodium salts.

158. Add perchloric acid: a white crystalline ppt.

159. Introduce a platinum wire, to which a portion of the substance adheres, into the colorless flame of a Bunsen burner, and observe the flame through a bit of blue glass: the flame is colored violet.

N. B.—The above reactions show the presence of potassium, which may be present as the hydrate, or as one of the salts of the metal. In cases of fatal corrosion by KHO, or of poisoning by the K salts, a quantitative determination is necessary.

Caustic Soda—Sodium Hydrate. NaHO.

In testing for the sodium compounds, the solutions must be concentrated.

160. Add hydrofluosilicic acid: a white gelatinous ppt.

161. Dissolve some potassium pyroantimoniate in boiling water, and filter. Add a portion of the filtrate to the

liquid under examination (which must not contain metals
other than K and Li): a white ppt., which becomes crystalline.

162. Colors the Bunsen flame yellow. Owing to its
great delicacy, this test is of little value in ordinary work,
as all substances examined contain sufficient Na to color
the flame.

N. B.—The above reactions merely indicate the presence
of Na without determining the form of combination. In
cases of fatal corrosion by NaHO, a quantitative analysis is
called for.

Aqua Ammoniæ—Ammonium Hydrate. NH_4HO.

163. The characteristic odor of ammonia is given off
by the hydrate and carbonate, but not by other ammoniacal salts.

164. Heat the liquid. Hold over it a strip of moistened
red litmus paper; it turns blue. Now hold over the heated
liquid a glass rod moistened with HCl; white fumes are
given off. These appearances are produced with ammoniacal salts other than the carbonate only if the liquids have
been previously rendered alkaline with KHO.

165. With HCl and $PtCl_4$: a yellow crystalline ppt. A
similar ppt. with K salts.

166. Dissolve chloride of lime and carbolic acid in
water, filter; add the liquid to be tested to the filtrate: a
green color.

167. Antidotes to the Alkalies.—Dilute vinegar
or lemon juice, milk. Under no circumstances should the
stomach-pump be used. Opium to allay pain. Nutritive
enemata if necessary.

METALLIC POISONS.

168. Preliminary to the separation of mineral poisons
from the tissues or contents of the stomach, the organic

matter must be destroyed by oxidation, as completely as is possible, without risk of loss of the substances sought for. This is best effected by the method of Frezenius and Von Babo. The substances under examination. hashed if solid, are diluted with water. About 50 cc. HCl* and a small quantity of powered potassium chlorate are added, and the whole heated over the water-bath. Small portions of $KClO_3$, and more HCl, *if necessary*, are added from time to time, until the mass is reduced to a yellow liquid on whose surface floats a layer of oil. The decomposition is accelerated by stirring and crushing any solid particles with the flattened end of a glass rod. When decomposition is complete, the liquid is allowed to cool, and filtered. If the filtrate smell of Cl, it is heated over the water-bath and treated with CO_2 until free of Cl. The liquid is now treated with H_2S for periods of an hour at a time, at intervals of twelve hours during two or three days; the flask containing it being kept corked during the intervals. A ppt. is always formed if a portion of the body has been operated on. This ppt. is collected on a filter and the filtrate (C) preserved. The ppt. is slightly washed and treated on the filter with yellow NH_4HS, concentrated at first. afterward dilute, so long as anything is dissolved. Any solid matter remaining undissolved on the filter is subsequently examined (B). The filtrate is evaporated to dryness in a porcelain capsule. To the residue 25 cc. H_2O, 2 cc. HCl, and a little $KClO_3$ are added, and the whole heated over the water-bath. The liquid is stirred until hot, small quantities of $KClO_3$ are added from time to time, and the mixture stirred until all is dissolved, except a little sulphur. The liquid is then treated with CO_2 over the water-bath till

* Hydrochloric acid cannot be bought sufficiently pure for this purpose. It must be made in the laboratory from pure NaCl and arsenic free H_2SO_4.

free of Cl, filtered, cooled, and treated with H_2S as before. The ppt. is collected on a filter and washed with H_2O, containing a little H_2S, until the washings, after boiling with HNO_3, fail to give *any* cloudiness with $AgNO_3$. The ppt. is now dissolved off the filter with NH_4HS, the solution evaporated in a porcelain capsule, the residue moistened with fuming HNO_3, dried over the water-bath, moistened with H_2O and dried two or three times, and finally fused with a mixture of $NaNO_3$ and Na_2CO_3 until it is colorless, or only contains a black powder. After cooling, the fused mass is dissolved in H_2O, treated with CO_2, and the solution filtered; the ppt., if any, on the filter (A) is examined as below. The filtrate is treated with excess of H_2SO_4 and heated, first over the water-bath, and afterwards at a higher temperature, until copious white fumes are given off; after cooling, the residue is examined for ARSENIC.

The ppt. A contains any Sb, Sn, or Cu (part) that may have been present. It is first, if black, treated with hot dil. HNO_3. The soln. so obtained is examined for COPPER. If the soln. from which it was filtered was turbid from the presence of a white material, the filter with adherent matter, insoluble in dil. HNO_3, after having been washed, is dried and burnt in a porcelain crucible, a small quantity of KCN is added to the ash, and the mixture fused for about ten minutes. After cooling, the contents of the crucible are treated with H_2O, and washed with H_2O by decantation, so long as anything is dissolved. The remaining metallic particles are treated with dil. HCl, the liquid separated, after warming on the water-bath, and tested for TIN. If any undissolved metallic particles remain, they are dissolved in hot concentrated HCl, and the soln. is tested for ANTIMONY.

If the portion B, insoluble in NH_4HS, be white, it

contains no poisonous metal. If it be colored, it is heated with HNO_3 so long as red fumes are given off, more HNO_3 being added if necessary, evaporated nearly to dryness, a little dil. H_2SO_4 added, allowed to stand for a time, and filtered. The filtrate is tested for BISMUTH and COPPER. The residue, if any, is treated with tartaric acid, and then with excess of NH_4HO, boiled, and filtered. The filtrate is tested for LEAD. The residue, if any, is dissolved in aqua regia, the soln. evaporated, the residue dissolved in H_2O, acidulated with HCl, and tested for MERCURY.

The liquid C contains any BARIUM, CHROMIUM, or ZINC that may have been present in the substances examined.

Arsenic. As.

169. Heat a small quantity As_2O_3 in a reduction tube.* Minute octahedral crystals of As_2O_3, which present brilliant reflections when the tube is rotated in sunlight, are deposited above the heated portion of the tube (Fig. 28, p. 58).

170. Heat a small quantity of Paris green in a reduction tube: crystals of As_2O_3 are formed, as in § 169.

171. Heat a small portion of elementary As in a long reduction tube: a brilliant steel-gray, brown, or black metallic-looking band is formed.

172. Cut off the bottom of the tube used in § 171; heat the band, holding the tube in an inclined position: the metallic band disappears, and above the point which it occupied, a crystalline sublimate of As_2O_3 is deposited.

173. Put a small quantity of As_2O_3 into a long reduction tube, and above it a splinter of charcoal. Heat the charcoal first, then the As_2O_3: a metallic band as in § 171 is

---

* A glass tube, 3–4 mm, in internal diameter and 8 cent. long, closed at one end.

formed. Cut off the bottom of the tube, and heat as in § 172: crystals of As_2O_3 are formed.

174. Acidulate soln. H_3AsO_3 with 2 gtt. HCl and pass H_2S through the soln.: a yellow ppt. of As_2S_3 is formed. Warm the contents of the tube, agitate, collect the ppt. on a filter, and wash. Divide the ppt. into four parts on four watch-glasses.

175. Add NH_4HS to one watch-glass: the ppt. dissolves.

176. Another portion of ppt. § 175 is treated with NH_4HO: it dissolves.

177. Another portion of ppt. § 175 is treated with HCl: it does not dissolve.

178. Mix the remaining portion, after drying, with potassium ferrocyanide, and heat a portion in a long reduction tube: a metallic band is formed. Cut off end of tube; heat as in § 172: crystals of As_2O_3.

179. To soln. H_3AsO_3 in a test-tube add KHO to alkaline reaction, and treat with H S: no ppt. is formed. Add HCl: a yellow ppt. is formed as in § 175.

180. Acidulate soln. H_3AsO_4 with HCl, and treat with H_2S: the liquid first turns yellow and cloudy, but the yellow ppt. of As_2S_3 only begins to form after a time.

181. Put 5 cc. H_2O into a porcelain capsule, add 1 gtt. NH_4HO, and then $CuSO_4$ until the ppt. formed no longer redissolves. To the liquid so obtained add about 1 cc. of the liquid under examination: a green ppt. Stir the mixture and transfer it in about equal portions to two test-tubes. To one tube add HNO_3: the ppt. dissolves, and the liquid becomes colorless. To the other test-tube add NH_4HO: the ppt. dissolves, forming a blue soln.

182. Put 5 cc. H_2O into a porcelain capsule; add 1 gtt. NH_4HO, and then $AgNO_3$ soln. until a permanent ppt. remains. Add 1 cc. H_3AsO_3 soln: a canary-yellow ppt. If the ppt. do not appear, test the reaction of the contents of the capsule, and render neutral by the *cautious* addition of very dil. HNO_3 or NH_4HO. Transfer to two test-tubes, and add HNO_3 to one, NH_4HO to the other: both clear to colorless solutions.

183. Repeat the test as in § 182, using a soln. of H_3AsO_4 in place of H_3AsO_3: a brick-red ppt., which also dissolves in HNO_3 and in NH_4HO.

184. *Reinsch's test.*—To 5 cc. in a test-tube add 0.5 cc. HCl and a slip of sheet Cu 2 mm. wide and 2 cent. long ; boil about five minutes, adding H_2O to supply loss by evaporation. If the Cu remain *perfectly* bright, the materials are pure; if the Cu become *even faintly* dimmed, the materials (Cu or HCl) are impure, and others must be substituted.

Having proven the purity of the reagents, put about 5 cc. of the liquid under examination into a test-tube. add 0.5 cc. HCl and a slip of Cu, and boil. The Cu becomes gray, then black. Remove the Cu, wash it in H_2O, dry between filter paper, taking care not to detach the black deposit. Place the Cu strip in and about 3 cent. from one end of a glass tube about 3 mm. in internal diameter and 15 cent. long. Warm the tube cautiously, holding it at an angle of 45° to the horizontal, until all moisture is driven off, then hold the tube at the same angle in the flame, so that the Cu is heated to bright redness. A white band is formed above the point at which the Cu was heated. Rotate the tube in the sunlight; brilliant, diamond-like reflections are seen. Examine the white band with a magnifier; it is found to consist of octahedral crystals of As_2O_3 (Fig. 28) (see §§ 192, 207, 237).

185. *Marsh's test.*—Place some granulated zinc in a flask of 100 cc. capacity; fit the cork carrying a funnel tube and right-angled tube (*a*, Fig. 29). Connect the right-angle tube with the drying tube *b*, filled with fragments of CaCl₂ or CaO between loose plugs of cotton, and connect this in turn with the Bohemian tube *c*. Pour dil. H_2SO_4 through the funnel tube in small quantities at a time. so

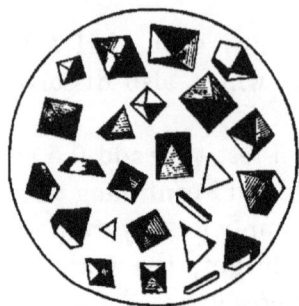

FIG. 28.

that a moderate evolution of H_2 results. After twenty minutes, light the burner *d*, and the gas escaping at *e*, and, after another half-hour, examine the tube at *c*. If the tube be *perfectly clean*, the Zn and H_2SO_4 are free from arsenic; but if any deposit have formed at *c*, the reagents contain As and must be discarded.

Having thus proved the purity of the chemicals, introduce the liquid to be tested, strongly acidulated with

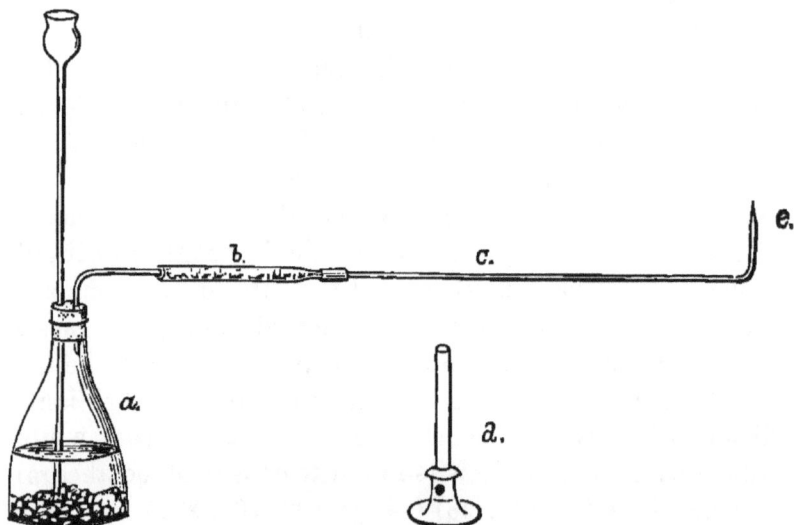

FIG. 29.

H_2SO_4, through the funnel tube in small portions at a time, and at such a rate that two hours would be consumed in

adding 25 cc. If As be present, a black or brown, single
or double, metallic "mirror" is produced at c. After the
mirror has become quite distinct, the tube c may be dis-
connected from b, another tube fitted, and a second mirror
collected. Now extinguish the burner, and hold a short
section (about two cent.), cut from the bottom of a test-
tube, over the flame at e, and, after a few moments, remove and examine it. If As be present in sufficient quantity, the brilliant octahedral crystals of As_2O_3 will be
found deposited on the glass. Next hold the cover of a
porcelain crucible *in* the flame at e for a short time; a
brown stain is formed on the porcelain. Collect several
similar stains on porcelain, and examine them as follows:
1. Moisten one with sodium hypochlorite soln.; it dissolves
instantly. 2. Moisten with NH_4HS soln. and warm; it
dissolves slowly. 3. Evaporate the soln. 2 to dryness; a
yellow residue remains. 4. Obtain three residues as in 3.
Moisten one with NH_4HO, the other with HCl; the former
dissolves, the latter does not. 5. Moisten the third residue 4 with HNO_3; it dissolves. Evaporate to dryness; a
white residue remains. Moisten with $AgNO_3$ soln.; it
turns brick-red.

Lastly, take one of the tubes c in which a mirror has
been formed, cut off the bent portion, and, holding the tube
at an angle of 45° to the horizontal, cautiously heat the
mirror: it disappears, and above it a white ring is deposited, consisting of the brilliant octahedral crystals of
As_2O_3.

Marsh's test is the most delicate and reliable of the tests
for arsenic. Great caution is, however, required that the
chemicals used do not themselves contain arsenic.

186. ANTIDOTES.—Emetics, stomach-pump, dialyzed
iron, ferric hydrate. The last-named is made by adding
excess of aqua ammoniæ to liq. ferri tersulphatis, collecting

the ppt. in a piece of muslin, and washing at the tap until the washings do not smell of ammonia. It is to be given moist, and in quantities at least twenty times as great as the amount of As_2O_3 to be neutralized.

Antimony. Sb.

187. To 5 cc. of the soln. to be tested add 2 gtt. HCl: a white ppt. of Sb_2O_3, if the soln. be not too dilute. Continue the addition of HCl: the ppt. redissolves.

188. Treat the soln. from § 187 with H_2S: an orange-red ppt. Collect the ppt. on a filter; wash with H_2O and place portions in three test-tubes.

189. Add NH_4HS to a portion of the ppt. from § 188: it dissolves.

190. Add NH_4HO to a portion of the ppt. from § 188: it does not dissolve.

191. Add HCl to a portion of the ppt. from § 188, and warm: it dissolves.

192. Apply *Reinsch's test* as directed in § 184; a stain, like that produced by arsenic, is formed upon the Cu. Upon heating the Cu in the glass tube, a white band is produced as in the case of As, but this band *consists of amorphous material* (Sb_2O_3). *not of crystals.*

193. Apply *Marsh's test* as directed in § 185. A metallic mirror, closely resembling that consisting of As, is formed in the tube *c*, fig. 29; it differs, however, from the arsenical mirror in being situated nearer to the heated portion of the tube, in disappearing less rapidly when heated in the tube through which a current of air is passing, and in yielding an *amorphous,* in place of a crystalline sublimate when so heated. The stains produced on porcelain differ from those consisting of As, in that: 1. They are insoluble in sodium hypochlorite soln. 2. They dissolve quickly in NH_4HS. 3. The residue of evaporation of the soln. from 2 is orange-red in color, is soluble in warm HCl, and insoluble in NH_4HO. 4. The residue of evaporation of the soln. from 2, when dissolved in warm HNO_3 and evaporated, leaves a white residue which does not become colored on addition of $AgNO_3$.

N. B.—If the method described in § 168 have been followed, As and Sb will have been separated, the latter having been precipitated from the soln. before the liquid is introduced into the Marsh apparatus, and, consequently, the two elements cannot be mistaken for one another.

194. ANTIDOTES.—Warm water to produce emesis if it have not occurred, stomach-pump, tannin (decoction of oak bark, cinchona, nutgalls, tea).

Bismuth. Bi.

195. Dissolve Bi in HNO_3, and dissolve the white, crystalline residue in dil. HCl. Divide the soln. into two parts.

196. Treat half the soln. obtained in § 195 with H_2S, a brownish-black ppt. is formed. Divide the liquid and suspended ppt. into three portions in three test-tubes.

197. To one test-tube, § 196, add NH_4HS: the ppt. does not dissolve.

198. To another test-tube, § 196, add KHO; the ppt. does not dissolve.

199. To another test-tube, § 196, add, after decanting as much as possible, HNO_3: the ppt. dissolves.

200. Add NH_4HS to a portion of the second half of the soln., § 195: a brownish-black ppt., having the same properties as that formed in § 196, is formed.

201. Add a small portion of the soln., § 195, to a large quantity of H_2O; a milkiness is produced (if the amount of HCl in the soln. be not too great), which clears on addition of HCl and application of heat.

202. Add KHO, NaHO, or NH₄HO to a portion of soln., § 195: a white ppt.

203. Add strong sodium acetate soln. to part of soln., § 195, and then⁻ potassium chromate soln.: a yellow, flocculent ppt. Divide the ppt. into two parts in two test-tubes.

204. To one test-tube, § 203, add KHO: the ppt. does not dissolve.

205. To the other test-tube, § 203, add HNO_3 in excess: the ppt. dissolves.

206. Add potassium ferrocyanide soln. to part of soln., § 195: a yellowish ppt., insoluble in HCl.

207. When *Reinsch's test* is applied to a soln. containing Bi, the Cu becomes stained as with As and Sb, but no sublimate is formed when it is heated in the glass tube.

Copper. Cu.

208. Treat with H_2S: brownish-black ppt. Collect the ppt. on a filter, and wash with H_2O containing H_2S, keeping the funnel covered with a glass plate. Place some of the ppt. in four test-tubes.

Add KHO to a portion of ppt.: it does not dissolve.
Add NH_4HS to a part of ppt.: it does not dissolve.
Boil part of ppt. with dil. H_2SO_4: it does not dissolve.
Boil part of ppt. with dil. HNO_3: it dissolves.

209. Add KHO: a pale blue ppt. Boil the liquid: the ppt. contracts and turns black.

210. Add 2 gtt. dil. NH_4HO: a greenish-blue ppt. Add a further quantity of NH_4HO: the ppt. dissolves, forming a dark-blue soln.

211. Add potassium ferrocyanide soln: a brown ppt. Add acetic acid: the ppt. does not dissolve.

212. Add a few gtt. H_2SO_4, and immerse in the soln. a piece of bright Fe wire: the wire is coated after a time with a non-adherent film of Cu.

213. Moisten a loop of Pt wire with the soln., and hold it in the lower portion of the Bunsen flame, which is then colored green.

214. ANTIDOTES.—Stomach-pump, albumen.

Lead. Pb.

215. Treat with H_2S: a black ppt. Wash the ppt. with H_2O, containing H_2S, and place portions of it in four test-tubes.

Add KHO to one test-tube: the ppt. does not dissolve.

Add NH_4HS to another test-tube: the ppt. does not dissolve.

Add dil. HNO_3 to another test-tube, and boil: the ppt. dissolves.

Add strong HNO_3 to another test-tube, and boil: the black color of the ppt. is discharged, and a white insoluble material remains. The PbS has been oxidized to $PbSO_4$.

216. Add HCl: a white ppt., if the soln. be not too dilute. Heat the liquid : the ppt. dissolves. Allow the liquid to cool: the $PbCl_2$ separates in crystals.

217. Add NH_4HO: a white ppt., insoluble in excess.

218. Add KHO: a white ppt. Add excess KHO and heat: the ppt. dissolves.

219. Add dil. H_2SO_4: a white ppt.

220. Add KI: a yellow ppt. Wash the ppt., suspend portion in H_2O; boil, and filter hot: on cooling, the soln. deposits brilliant yellow crystals.

221. Add potassium chromate: a yellow ppt. Collect the ppt., wash, and place portions in two test-tubes.

To one test-tube add KHO: the ppt. dissolves.

To the other test-tube add acetic acid: the ppt. does not dissolve.

222. Suspend a piece of Zn. in the soln.: crystals of metallic lead separate after a time.

223. ANTIDOTES.—Magnesium or sodium sulphate; stomach-pump; emetics.

Mercury. Hg.

MERCUROUS (Hg₂).

224. Heat a small quantity of calomel in a reduction tube: it does not fuse, but turns yellow and sublimes.

225. Add HCl to soln. $Hg_2(NO_3)_2$: a white ppt. Add NH_4HO: the ppt. does not dissolve, but turns black.

226. Add NH_4HO to soln. $Hg_2(NO_3)_2$: a black ppt., insol. in excess.

227. Add KHO to soln. $Hg_2(NO_3)_2$: a black ppt., insol. in excess.

228. Add KI to soln. $Hg_2(NO_3)_2$, without excess of HNO_3: a greenish ppt.

MERCURIC. Hg.

229. Heat a small portion of corrosive sublimate in a reduction tube: it turns yellowish, fuses, and sublimes.

230. Add HCl to soln. $HgCl_2$: no ppt. is formed.

231. Add NH_4HO: a white ppt., sol. in solns. of NH_4 salts.

232. Add KHO: a yellow ppt., insol. in excess.

233. Add 2 gtt. KI to soln. $HgCl_2$: a salmon colored ppt., which turns red rapidly. Add excess KI: the ppt. dissolves, forming a colorless soln.

MERCUROUS AND MERCURIC.

234. Treat with H_2S: a ppt., which is first white, then orange, then brown, and finally black. Collect the ppt.

on a filter, wash until the washings are free from Cl, and place portions of the ppt. in three test-tubes.

Add strong HCl to one test-tube, and boil: the ppt. does not dissolve.

Add strong HNO_3 to another test-tube, and boil: the ppt. does not dissolve.

Mix the contents of the two tubes, and heat: the ppt. dissolves.

Add NH_4HS to the remaining tube, and warm: the ppt. does not dissolve.

235. Dissolve a fragment of Sn in HCl with the aid of heat. Add a few gtt. of this soln. to 1 cc. soln. $HgCl_2$: a white ppt. Add more $SnCl_2$ soln.: the ppt. turns gray. Boil the liquid, decant as much of the liquid from the ppt. as possible, add HCl to the ppt., and boil: the ppt. unites into globules of metallic Hg.

236. Pour dil. HNO_3 on a copper cent. When the Cu has become bright, pour off the acid, wash the coin with water, and immerse it in soln. $HgCl_2$, acidulated with HCl: after a time the Cu is covered with a gray film. Rub the surface of the coin with the finger: it assumes a silvery lustre.

237. Apply *Reinsch's test* to a soln. of $HgCl_2$: the Cu is stained as with As, Sb, and Bi, but when heated in the glass tube it yields a sublimate consisting of minute globules of Hg.

238. Immerse a bar of Zn, around which a strip of dentist's gold foil has been wound, so as to leave exposed alternate surfaces of Zn and Au, in dil. soln. $HgCl_2$, acidulated with HCl. The Au is covered with a silvery film and, when heated in a glass tube, yields a sublimate consisting of globules of Hg.

239. ANTIDOTES.—White of egg; followed in a few moments by an emetic, or stomach-pump.

Barium. Ba.

240. With $(NH_4)_2CO_3$, a white ppt., sol. in acids.

241. With dil. H_2SO_4, or $CaSO_4$ soln., a white ppt., insol. in acids.

242. With $HC_2H_3O_2$ and K_2CrO_4, a yellow ppt., sol. in warm $HC_2H_3O_2$.

243. On Pt wire, colors Bunsen flame yellowish-green.

244. ANTIDOTES.—Magnesium or sodium sulphate.

Zinc. Zn.

245. Add NH_4Cl and NH_4HO to alkaline reaction, and treat with H_2S: a white ppt. Transfer the liquid and suspended ppt. to three test-tubes.

To one tube add NH_4HS: the ppt. does not dissolve.

To another tube add $HC_2H_3O_2$: the ppt. does not dissolve.

To the third add HCl: the ppt. dissolves.

246. Add KHO in small quantity: a white ppt. Add excess of KHO: the ppt. dissolves. Add H_2O and boil: a white ppt. again separates.

247. Add potassium ferrocyanide: a white ppt., insol. in HCl.

248. ANTIDOTES.—Milk, white of egg, tea, tannin.

249. In this class are included the alkaloids, glucosides, and vegetable acids. Their separation from organic mixtures, contents of stomach, organs, etc., is best effected by a combination of the Stas-Otto and Dragendorff methods. The substances to be examined, hashed if solid, are placed in a flask and covered with twice their weight of alcohol,* alcoholic solution of tartaric acid is then added, during agitation, until the contents of the flask are distinctly acid. The mouth of the flask is closed with a cork, through which passes a glass-tube of 8 mm. internal diameter and about a meter long, open at both ends, and the flask warmed over the water-bath about two hours. The contents of the flask are allowed to cool, filtered through a filter moistened with alcohol, and the insol. portion washed with alcohol. The alcoholic filtrate and washings are evaporated in a porcelain capsule at a temperature of 35° C., until the alcohol is removed. The aqueous liquid remaining is cooled, filtered, and the filtrate evaporated to the consistence of syrup. To the syrupy residue a few gtt. absolute alcohol are added and the mixture thoroughly stirred. The addition of absolute alcohol in small portions, during constant stirring, is continued so long as any precipitate is formed. The alcoholic liquid is filtered off and the residue washed with alcohol. The filtrate and washings are evaporated to the consistence of

---

* Alcohol for this purpose must be purified by dissolving in it tartaric acid to strongly acid reaction, and distilling over the water-bath.

syrup, and the residue dissolved in H_2O. The distinctly
acid aqueous soln. is transferred to a bulb funnel (Fig. 30)
in which it is agitated with different solvents as follows:

The acid, aqueous liquid is agitated with petroleum
ether, the ethereal layer separated, and evaporated. This
treatment, like all of the subsequent agitations, is repeated
so long as the solvent dissolves anything. The petroleum
ether leaves a residue, Residue I., which contains
principally fatty, resinous, and pigmentary substances.

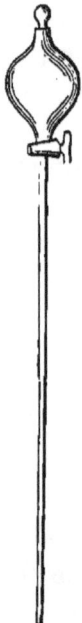

The acid, aqueous liquid is next agitated with
benzol, which is evaporated in several watch glasses.
This, Residue II., may contain colchicin, digita-
lin, and small quantities of veratrine and physostigmine.

The acid, aqueous liquid is then agitated with
chloroform, which is evaporated on watch glasses,
yielding Residue III., which may contain picro-
toxin and digitalëin and traces of brucine, narcotine, physostigmine, and veratrine.

The acid, aqueous liquid is again agitated with
petroleum ether to remove $CHCl_3$, the ether separated, and the aqueous liquid rendered alkaline
with NH_4HO.

The alkaline, aqueous liquid is agitated with
petroleum ether, which, on separation and evaporation in watch glasses, leaves Residue IV.,
which may contain coniïne and nicotine, and traces of
brucine, strychnine, and veratrine.

Fig. 30.

The alkaline, aqueous liquid is next agitated with benzol, which is evaporated, yielding Residue V., in which
atropine, hyoscyamine, narcotine, strychnine, aconitine,
brucine, physostigmine, and veratrine may be found.

The alkaline, aqueous liquid is then agitated with chloroform, which, on evaporation, leaves Residue VI., which may contain the opium alkaloids in small quantity.

The alkaline, aqueous liquid is lastly agitated with amylic alcohol, from which Residue VII., in which morphine will be found if present in the substances examined, is obtained by evaporation.

Finally, curarine, if present, will remain in the aqueous liquid, which may also contain oxalic acid.

General Reactions of Alkaloids.

250. Add to an acidulated soln. of an alkaloid a soln. of potassium iodhydrargyrate, made by dissolving 13.546 gms. $HgCl_2$ and 49.8 gms. KI in 1 L. H_2O; a white or yellow ppt.

N. B.—This reaction, like the subsequent ones, is best performed by placing a drop of the liquid under examination and one of the reagent near each other on a slip of black glass and bringing the two together with a pointed glass rod.

251. Add to an acidulated soln. of an alkaloid, a soln. of phosphomolybdic acid: a white or yellow ppt.

252. Add to an acidulated soln. of an alkaloid, soln. of phosphotungstic acid: a white, flocculent ppt.

253. The following reagents also produce ppts. in faintly acidulated solns. of alkaloids: Iodine in potassium iodide, brown; tannin, white or yellow; platinic chloride, yellowish, usually becoming crystalline; auric chloride, yellowish; phosphoantimonic acid, white; iodide of potassium and iodide of cadmium, white or yellow; picric acid, yellow.

Morphine.

254. Moisten a crystal with HNO_3: a red color, changing to yellow.

255. Moisten with H_2SO_4: the alkaloid dissolves, forming a colorless soln. Let stand twenty-four hours, and add a trace of HNO_3: the liquid turns pink. Warm, cool, dilute with H_2O and add a small crystal of potassium dichromate: a mahogany color.

256. Dissolve a few crystals of iodic acid in H_2O, and shake a part of the soln. with $CHCl_3$, the latter should not be colored.

Add to a soln. of a morphine salt a few gtt. of the iodic acid soln. and agitate: the liquid assumes a yellow color. Add a few gtt. $CHCl_3$, and agitate: the $CHCl_3$ which separates at the bottom is colored violet. Float some dil. NH_4HO on the surface of the liquid: the test-tube will contain different colored layers; violet below, then yellow, dark yellow or brown, and faintly yellowish.

257. Moisten a crystal of morphine, or add to a neutral soln. of one of its salts, a neutral soln. of Fe_2Cl_6: a blue color.

258. To a crystal of morphine add a soln. of molybdic acid in H_2SO_4 (Fröhde's reagent): a violet color, changing to blue, dirty green, and faint pink. Water discharges the color.

259. Add NH_4HO to $AgNO_3$ soln. until the ppt. begins to remain undissolved, filter, add soln. of a morphine salt and warm: a gray ppt. Filter off the liquid and add to it HNO_3: a red or pink color.

260. ANTIDOTES.—Stomach-pump, wash out stomach with H_2O, holding powdered charcoal in suspension, or with infusion of tea, $ZnSO_4$. Keep patient awake. Atropine?

Meconic Acid.

261. To portions of the acid in three watch glasses add Fe_2Cl_6 soln: a red color is produced. To one watch glass add dil. HCl: the color is not discharged. To the second watch glass add $HgCl_2$ soln.: the color is not discharged.

To the third watch glass add sodium hypochlorite soln.: the color is discharged.

262. Add Fe_2Cl_6 soln. to a sulphocyanate in a watch glass: a red color, similar to that with meconic acid, is produced. Add $HgCl_2$ soln.: the color is discharged.

Strychnine.

263. Place a minute drop of a soln. of a strychnine salt on the tongue: a persistent, intensely bitter taste.

264. Add H_2SO_4: the alkaloid (or its salts) dissolves, forming a colorless soln. Draw through the soln. a fragment of a crystal of potassium dichromate: it is followed by a streak of color; at first blue (very transitory and frequently not observed), then a brilliant violet, which slowly changes to rose pink, and finally to yellow.

265. Evaporate a drop of soln. of a strychnine salt on a slip of Pt. foil, moisten the residue with concentrated H_2SO_4, connect the foil with the + pole of a Grove cell, and bring a Pt. wire, connected with the — pole in contact with the surface of the acid: a violet color on the surface of the foil.

266. Moisten a fragment of strychnine with a soln. of iodic acid in H_2SO_4: a yellow color, changing to brick-red and then to violet-red.

267. Let an assistant hold a small frog by the hind legs. Raise the skin of the back at the root of the legs with a forceps, make a small incision with a scissors and allow a few gtt. of a very dilute soln. of a salt of strychnine to flow into the lymph pouch. Place the frog under a glass shade: within ten minutes the animal has violent tetanic spasms, with opisthotonos or emprosthotonos, increasing in frequency, and provoked on the slightest touch, or by blowing upon the surface.

268. Add a few gtt. of a dil. soln. of potassium dichromate to a soln. of a strychnine salt: a yellow, crystalline ppt. Collect the ppt. and moisten it with conc. H_2SO_4: a play of colors as in § 264.

269. ANTIDOTES.—Stomach-pump, wash out stomach with infusion of tea. Chloroform, chloral.

Atropine.

270. Dissolve a fragment of potassium dichromate in a few gtt. H_2SO_4, warm, add a fragment of atropine and two gtt. H_2O, and stir: an odor resembling that of orange blossoms.

271. Drop a few gtt. of a dil. soln. of a salt of atropine into the inner canthus of the eye of a cat, after a few moments hold the animal so that the light falls equally upon both eyes: the pupil of the eye operated upon is widely dilated.

272. Add a five-per-cent solution of $HgCl_2$ in fifty per cent C_2H_6O, and warm gently; a brick-red ppt.

273. Dissolve the substance to be tested in alcohol. Heat some mercuric cyanide in a short test-tube, fitted with a cork and bent glass tube. Pass the gas evolved from the $Hg(CN)_2$ into the alcoholic soln.: it assumes a blood-red color.

274. Moisten the solid alkaloid with conc. HNO_3, dry on the water-bath, cool, add a drop of an alcoholic soln. of KHO: a violet color passing to a brilliant red.

275. ANTIDOTES.—Emetics, stomach-pump, wash out stomach with infusion of tea. Morphine?

Oxalic Acid.

276. Add NH_4HO to neutral or faintly alkaline reaction, then a soln. of $CaCl_2$: a white ppt. Add HCl: the ppt. dissolves.

277. Add $AgNO_3$: a white ppt. Boil the liquid: the

ppt. does not darken. Divide the ppt. and liquid into two portions; to one add HNO_3, to the other NH_4HO: the ppt. in each dissolves.

278. Add $Pb(C_2H_3O_2)_2$: a white ppt. if the soln. be not too dilute. Divide the liquid and ppt. into two parts, to one add HNO_3: the ppt. dissolves; to the other add $HC_2H_3O_2$: the ppt. does not dissolve.

279. ANTIDOTES.—Slacked lime, magnesia usta, suspended in a *small quantity* of water. Give as little liquid as possible, and do not use stomach-pump if symptoms of corrosion are observed.

INDEX.

www.ingramcontent.com/pod-product-compliance
Lightning Source LLC
Chambersburg PA
CBHW021958190326
41519CB00010B/1315